Charity's
Sister

Charity's Sister

~†~

The story of
Sister Mary Joaquin Bitler, SC

Mari Graña

SUNSTONE
PRESS

SANTA FE

Sunstone books may be purchased for educational, business, or sales promotional use.
For information please write: Special Markets Department, Sunstone Press,
P.O. Box 2321, Santa Fe, New Mexico 87504-2321.

Book and Cover design ~ Vicki Ahl
Body typeface ~ Minion Pro
Printed on acid free paper

Library of Congress Cataloging-in-Publication Data

Graña, Mari, 1936-
  Charity's sister : the story of Sister Mary Joaquin Bitler, SC / by Mari Graña.
      p. ; cm.
  Includes bibliographical references.
  ISBN 978-0-86534-777-9 (softcover : alk. paper)
  1. Bitler, Mary Joaquin, 1922-2003. 2. Nurses--New Mexico--Biography. 3. Catholic
hospitals--New Mexico. I. Title.
  [DNLM: 1. Bitler, Mary Joaquin, 1922-2003. 2. Nurses--Mexico--Biography.
3. Nurses--New Mexico--Biography. 4. Catholicism--Mexico--Biography.
5. Catholicism--New Mexico--Biography. 6. Hospitals, Religious--Mexico--Biography.
7. Hospitals, Religious--New Mexico--Biography. 8. Missions and Missionaries--Mexico-
-Biography. 9. Missions and Missionaries--New Mexico--Biography. WZ 100]
  RT37.B58G73 2010
  610.73092--dc22
  [B]

                              2010033063

Published in

WWW.SUNSTONEPRESS.COM
SUNSTONE PRESS / POST OFFICE BOX 2321 / SANTA FE, NM 87504-2321 /USA
(505) 988-4418 / ORDERS ONLY (800) 243-5644 / FAX (505) 988-1025

*For every force charged by God…
with some business is an angel
put in charge.*
—Moses Maimonides (1135–1204)

~✝~

In memory of Sister of Charity Mary Joaquin Bitler, who dedicated her life to serving the sick and the poor

Contents

≈†≈

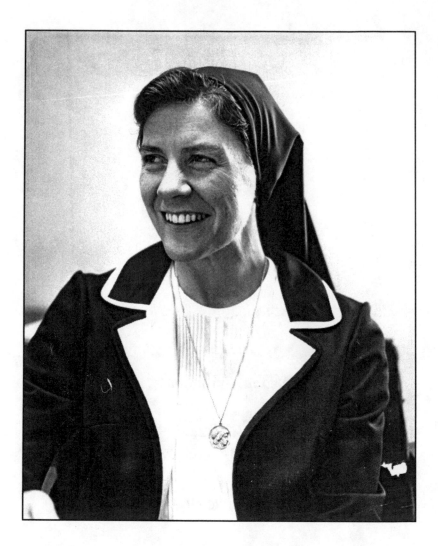

Sister Mary Joachim Bitler, 1965.
Photograph: Deborah Douglas collection.

Part I

~†~

St. Vincent Hospital.
Santa Fe, New Mexico

The thing that makes us different from other hospitals is our commitment to the whole person. To us, it's a little more than just putting bones back together.
—Sister Mary Joachim

1

~†~

When Sister Mary Joachim Bitler SC was sent by the Cincinnati Order of the Sisters of Charity to be Supervisor of Nursing at St. Vincent Hospital in Santa Fe, New Mexico, the young nurse was shocked at the backwardness of the institution. It was 1951, and Sister Mary Joachim had just finished four years as the Director of Nursing at Good Samaritan Hospital in Dayton, Ohio. "Good Sam," as local residents affectionately called the Dayton hospital, enjoyed the latest in equipment and advanced medical procedures. In contrast, Santa Fe's only hospital, built in 1910 and serving not only the city and county, but also much of the entire northern region of the state, was run, in the new nurse's words, on "nerve and hope."[1]

In 1951 St. Vincent Hospital was housed in the third hospital building constructed by the Sisters of Charity since their arrival in the wild west of New Mexico Territory in 1865. Once the Civil War ended, Jean-Baptiste Lamy, Bishop of Santa Fe, wrote Archbishop Purcell in Cincinnati, asking him to contact the Sisters of Charity—a Cincinnati Order of religious women dedicated to teaching, nursing, and service to the poor—and ask the sisters to send nurses to start a hospital in Santa Fe. Lamy, a transplant from France, had arrived in the territorial capital in 1851, not long after the United States had claimed New Mexico under the

Treaty of Guadalupe Hidalgo at the end of the Mexican-American War. At the time, New Mexico territory extended to what is now Arizona and southern parts of Colorado, Utah, and Nevada.

The French bishop was appalled at the poverty and ignorance in the area and the religious and racial prejudices—Anglos against Spanish and Indians, Spanish against Anglos and Indians, and Indians frequently attacking both. There were not yet any formal schools, no hospitals or orphanages or other institutions of civilization other than the Church— and the Church, prior to Lamy's arrival, had suffered the decadence of isolation, both geographically and from the secular policies of the Mexican government.[2] In addition to the bishop's attempts to bring a strict order to the religious life of the remote area and stamp out what he felt was the questionable morality of some of the New Mexican priests, he also wanted to improve the health and educational conditions of the mostly Spanish-speaking population of his new diocese.

The Cincinnati sisters sent four women, two of whom had been nurses during the Civil War, none of whom spoke Spanish. Traveling by boat, train, and finally stagecoach, a three-week journey, the easterners found a Santa Fe composed mainly of small adobe houses with dirt floors, tiny windows, and covered with flat, dirt roofs. Bishop Lamy had acquired land and a few adobe hovels behind the parish church of St. Francis—later to be transformed into his French-style neo-Romanesque cathedral—with three thousand dollars, bequeathed to him by the French priest he had installed in the town of Mora. The priest had died of poison in the sacramental Communion wine, a fate purportedly intended for his associate, who had neglected to show up for Mass that day.

The first Santa Fe hospital was located in one of the bishop's hovels, an orphanage was located in another. Lamy gave up half of his mud-floored house to the sisters—the part in which the roof didn't leak. When it rained, the good bishop ate his dinner with an umbrella over his head. The sisters named their hospital after St. Vincent de Paul, the early 17th century emissary to the poor and the patron saint of the Sisters of Charity. No one knows for certain who the first patients in the sisters' new St.

Vincent Hospital were, but they may have been the two priests shot by an intruder who had entered Lamy's quarters demanding money. The thief was soon hauled off to jail, and with the sisters' care, the two men survived. At the sisters' orphanage, their first orphan was a Navajo baby girl found abandoned on a battlefield. Every Saturday the poor would come to the hospital for food, and daily the sisters visited the homes of the sick.

The little hospital was enlarged with volunteer labor and contributed materials. The territorial legislature allocated a hundred dollars a month to help the project. Noting that the new hospital would perhaps be a refuge for the beggars who had been harassing the townspeople for alms, the law required the sheriff to present all mendicants found in the public streets to the hospital—to take them in if sick, to send them to work for a living if not.[3] Other sources of funds came trickling in, some from the clergy, some from the soldiers stationed at Fort Marcy, some from grateful families of patients, and some gathered by the sisters from their begging trips. The sisters walked for miles around the region begging funds, especially from the mine owners in Cerrillos and Madrid, who on the whole were very generous. Supplies were donated from the Fort Marcy commissary. Nevertheless the little hospital was continuously in dire financial straits, as well as lacking space, since the sisters' policy was to help everyone—Protestant, Catholic, Jew, atheist, Indian, Spanish or Anglo—regardless of his or her ability to pay, a policy that continues to this day.[4] In 1876, Sister Blandina Segale addressed the lack of hospital space to accommodate the many charity cases in a novel and practical way: she moved the paying patients into private homes.

Sister Blandina recorded a now almost legendary event in her memoir, *At the End of the Santa Fe Trail*. The sister was called to treat one of Billy-the-Kid's accomplices who had been wounded in a gun battle. She did so, and the young outlaw survived. Later, when Sister Blandina learned that Billy's gang was proposing to scalp four physicians whom Billy felt had refused them aid, she talked them out of it. Later, when the gang was poised to attack a stagecoach on the road from Trinidad to

Santa Fe, Billy realized that one of the passengers was Sister Blandina. On recognizing her, Billy tipped his hat to her and called off his men. From then on, any stage carrying a Sister of Charity—clearly recognizable by the cap and long black habit—was off limits to the gang.[5]

By the late1870s, the little hospital was overflowing with miners hurt in mining accidents and railroad workers suffering from smashed limbs. Additionally, the mild, healthful climate of Santa Fe was becoming famous as a place of possible cure for a U.S. population suffering from malaria, as well as tuberculosis, pneumonia, and other respiratory diseases. At a time when most doctors in the West gained their knowledge either from reading a do-it-yourself book or by working with other doctors who had gained their knowledge from working with yet other doctors, the St. Vincent Hospital physician, Dr. Robert Longwill, had actually graduated from Philadelphia's Jefferson Medical College. Although Dr. Longwill's medical competence was acknowledged, he was also one of the leaders of the Santa Fe Ring—a group of nefarious Anglo lawyers and certain Spanish land-owning *ricos* intent on separating the extensive lands granted the people by the previous Spanish and Mexican governments from their unsuspecting owners. Hence Longwill's reputation was not conducive to confidence among many in need of his help. To his credit, however, he was instrumental in convincing the legislature to pass a bill regulating the practice of medicine in the territory.[6]

In 1880 a three-story building was erected under the supervision of Sister Blandina. The building had been intended for a school, but with the coming of the railroad, the more immediate need was to use it as a hospital. In 1883 the Sisters opened a new sanatorium, and a few years later, a new orphanage. But fire destroyed the sanatorium in 1896, the patients being quickly rescued, some moved to the orphanage, some to the hospital that had escaped the fire, and some to the private homes of concerned Santa Fe residents.

One of the many stories about the sisters' hospital recounts that Territorial Governor Miguel Otero and two companions, inebriated and with pockets flush with poker winnings from a night on the town, knocked on the hospital door in the early morning hours. Sister Victoria graciously took them in. Otero offered her $50 for her good services. One of his companions insisted Otero double the amount, and the third man insisted he double that. The governor and his friends departed the next day, but returned to add another $50, bringing the total to the hospital for the night's debauchery at $250.[7]

It wasn't until 1910 that a seventy-five-bed, $75,000 modern hospital was built, opening to great public fanfare and acclaim—a military band, a bazaar, and free dinners for the townspeople. Facing onto Palace Avenue, the new hospital contained electric lights, hot and cold running water, steam heat, an X-ray unit, a large operating room on the third floor, and an elevator that sometimes worked. When it didn't, the hospital staff had to carry their patients, strapped into chairs, up and down the three floors. When extra beds were available, the sisters took in visitors, and the hospital, said to have the best dining room in town, soon became a community center. Parties were thrown in the billiards room off the main lobby, and when the legislature was in session, poker games went on through the night.[8] A great sport for the children was to slide down the stair banisters. Years later, one Santa Fean remembered she and her friends making so much noise in the lobby that the sisters sent them all to play in the old sanitarium, where there were only two occupants at the time, both of whom were deaf.

One of the more notorious operations at the Santa Fe hospital was performed by Sister Mary de Sales, who later became the first woman MD in New Mexico Territory. Using a penknife and forceps, Sister Mary removed a stone from a miner's eye. The stone now rests in a glass case in the Sisters of Charity's Motherhouse in Cincinnati.[9]

This was the hospital to which, in 1951, Sister Mary Joachim was sent to serve as Superintendent of Nurses.

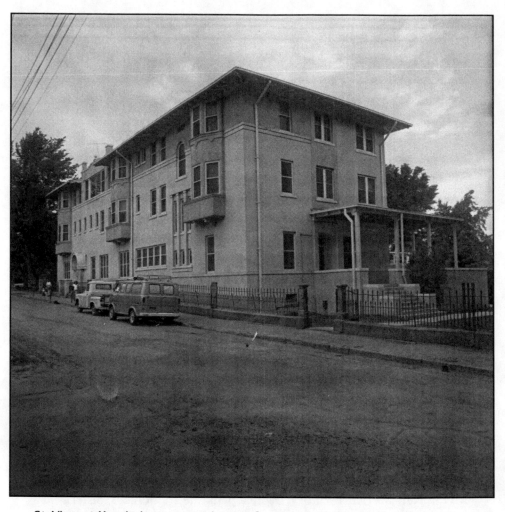

St. Vincent Hospital, constructed 1910. Converted 1953 to Marian Hall, a convent for the sister-nurses. Photograph, New Mexico History Museum Photo Archives no.117163

Sister Mary Joachim's tenure in the Santa Fe hospital lasted only eight months; she was soon transferred to the Sisters of Charity's hospital in Pueblo, Colorado, to take the position of Surgical Supervisor. A few years before Sister Joachim arrived at the Pueblo hospital, a fire had broken out in the basement of the sixty-three-year-old building, resulting in the destruction of a whole wing and consequently the loss of several beds. Discussions with the City of Pueblo regarding possible municipal financing to rebuild the damaged hospital, along with several fund drives, went on for the next several years. In 1948, however, another Pueblo hospital, the 46-year old Corwin Hospital, belonging to the Colorado Fuel and Iron Company, was put up for sale.[10] The initial asking price was a hundred thousand dollars. There were no takers. The CF&I, eager to get out of the hospital business, soon reduced the price to fifty thousand. There still were no takers, and the Company decided to turn the million-dollar facility over to the Sisters of Charity for a transfer fee of one dollar, and to throw in two thousand dollars for a convent chapel and several thousand for working capital. The sisters had to agree to maintain existing contracts, excluding the CIO United Steel Workers contract, to retain the name of Corwin for the hospital, and to maintain the hospital according to American Medical Association standards. The Cincinnati Order quickly agreed, and the deal seemed to the sisters a wonderful boon, bringing the number of their hospitals around the country to eleven. A boon—until two months after the agreement was signed. Suddenly, the nonprofessional Corwin employees walked out in a wildcat strike. The workers had voted affiliation with the CIO while the hospital was still owned by the CF&I, and they didn't see why a union should be permitted in an industrial hospital, but not in one run by a religious order. Fortunately there was no violence, and the worst damage was several flat tires from tacks set in the parking lot and some nasty words hurled at those who crossed the picket lines. There was a question as to the legality of the strike, since the recently enacted 1947 Taft-Hartley Act had specifically exempted nonprofit hospitals. Two sisters went immediately to Pittsburgh to see the president of the CIO, Phillip Murray. After a wait of several hours, the two were ushered into the president's office. Murray was accompanied by his legal counsel, Arthur J. Goldberg, the man who would later become a Supreme Court Justice. Murray and Goldberg listened to the sisters' story, then told them that there was little hope for a favorable solution.

At this, the women fell to their knees and began to pray aloud. To their surprise, the president and the lawyer joined them in their prayer, also kneeling on the floor. When the four had concluded their supplications to the Almighty, Murray agreed that a Catholic hospital was no place for a union, and after several phone calls, the strike was called off.[11]

Sister Mary Joachim was born Gina Rita Bitler on May 23, 1922, one of four children in a devout and musical family in Wapakoneta, a small town in Ohio. Gina's father, Milo Bitler, was an engineer, and her mother, Teresa della Chiesa, a renowned concert mezzo-soprano. Gina's grandfather, Giovanni della Chiesa, had played clarinet in John Phillips Souza's band and, prior to coming to America, oboe and clarinet in La Scala opera orchestra in Milan. There was always music in the Bitler home. Her grandfather gave music lessons, and Gina, as a little girl, would play quietly on the floor, listening to the lesson. One evening in 1932 when Gina was ten, her Uncle Don gave her a German Hohner harmonica and told her she must learn to play single notes on it, not just chords, which were easy. All through dinner that night and long after her bedtime, Gina practiced getting the harmonica to play single notes. Finally, after ignoring her mother's reprimands, she was threatened with "the paddle." But she finally managed to master the harmonica's single note scale. She kept that harmonica with her the rest of her life.

When Gina was twelve, her mother died. Her father married again, and Gina felt she could not live with her new stepmother. She moved in with her aunt, Nelle Kohler. Determined to become a concert musician, Gina studied piano all through high school, cleaning out coal furnaces in the winter and cutting her neighbors' lawns in the summer to pay for lessons. Babysitting was another money source, and years later she realized that one of her early charges was to become the first man on the moon—Wapakoneta's own Neil Armstrong.

Gina became accomplished as a pianist. At the same time she was influenced by her aunt Nelle, who was a nurse, and Gina could see that a nursing career offered financial security. After high school she worked as a dental assistant for a couple of years and then entered the school of nursing at Cincinnati's Good Samaritan Hospital. She hadn't given up her dream of becoming a professional musician, but her thinking was that a nursing profession would allow her security while she continued her music studies. Further, Cincinnati, being a music center, offered her the opportunity to attend the many operas and excellent concerts the city was famous for.

Gina's life was changed by her nursing studies at the hospital. She became interested in the Sisters of Charity, and one of the sisters, Sister Jean Clair Kenney, discussed with her the possibility of joining the Order. "I guess it would be dramatic to say that one single event was the deciding factor in my choice," the nun would recount years later, "but this was not the case. It was really very simple." After attending an outdoor performance of *Carmen* with Rise Stevens in the title role, Gina was thrilled by the music she had just heard, but was torn with indecision as to whether she should pursue a career in music or a career in nursing as a member of the Sisters of Charity.[12]

Gina was a devout Catholic, raised in a devout home. On her ride home after the opera that May evening, her decision suddenly became clear: she would become a postulate with the Sisters of Charity. Perhaps it was later that in her mind it was a simple decision. Gina had been greatly influenced by her aunt's dedication to helping the sick and the poor, and she was strongly attracted by Nelle Kohler's financial independence, her philosophy of helping others, and the patience and practicality of her aunt's life. It was the same philosophy of service to others that guided the Sisters of Charity as they sought to be the instruments of God's will. And joining the Order, the young woman reasoned, would not stop her from the concurrent development of her musical ambition.

In the fall of 1943, Gina Rita Bitler entered the Sisters of Charity. At the ceremony in which the novitiates were given their long black habit and cap, the women were also asked to choose the religious name they would answer to for the rest of their lives. One of Gina's fellow novitiates relates that everyone in the group assumed the new nun would choose the name Benedicta, since her mother, Teresa, had been a cousin of Pope Benedict XV, the pope in office during the Great War.[13] But instead, Gina declared her name would be Mary Joachim in honor of her reverence for the Virgin and in honor of her brother John—Joachim being a Hebrew form of John. Gina's novitiate sister was surprised, but since she had wanted the name Benedicta for herself, and Gina was ahead of her in line and hence stated her new name first, her sister and friend was able to take the name Benedicta. Sisters Mary Joachim and Benedicta both made their first commitment vows to the Sisters of Charity in 1945, and, after a month-long stay of discernment at the Cincinnati Motherhouse, made their perpetual vows together in 1950.[14] Once Gina had taken her new name, she was often called simply "Sister" or just "Joachim" by her friends and associates.[15] Many years later, when Sister Mary Joachim was asked what was the hardest thing for her to give up when she became a Sister of Charity, she answered without hesitation, "my dog and my bicycle."[16]

The Sisters of Charity sent the new nun for nurse's training at "Good Sam" in Dayton. She continued to pursue her musical interests, branching into arranging and composing as she continued her training. She graduated from the Dayton hospital's school of nursing in 1947. The following year she passed her examinations by the Ohio State Nursing Board and became a licensed Registered Nurse, remaining in Dayton as medical surgical supervisor. Three years later Sr. Mary Joachim, SC and RN was sent to St Vincent Hospital in Santa Fe to be Superintendent of Nursing.

2

~†~

Although Sister Mary Joachim's work as Superintendent of Nurses in the Santa Fe hospital lasted only a few months, she took time to attend concerts and to explore the museums and historical monuments of the capital city. She was fascinated by the melding of the city's diverse cultures—the Anglo, Indian, and Spanish—and appreciated the artistic creativity so evident around her. The art colony that was vibrant in Santa Fe at the time was mostly Anglo, but the population of the city and the surrounding region was still largely of Spanish and Mexican origin. Along with her music studies, she had also studied painting, and as an artist and a religious, she was drawn to the Hispanic Catholic folk art—paintings with gesso on wood, figure carvings depicting the saints and the Holy Family, and the crucifixes depicting Christ's agony that adorned the many little adobe churches of the area.

In addition to her love of the arts, and under the influence of her engineer father, she had excelled in math, chemistry and physics during her school years. Her knowledge of math proved helpful in the more bureaucratic aspects of nursing, and particularly later in her career, juggling the internal balancings of a hospital budget. She loved to swim, and became a Red Cross safety instructor, keeping her instructor's certificate current for many years. Swimming gave her great joy and relaxation, especially after long hours on the nursing floor.

When, in 1952, the Sisters of Charity called Sister Joachim to leave Santa Fe and go to the Corwin Hospital—later named St-Mary-Corwin—in Pueblo, she hoped someday to be able to return. In Colorado, her work as head of surgical nursing was even more demanding than in Santa Fe, and she had little time to continue her artistic interests. The mangled bodies that were brought into the hospital from industrial accidents in the steel mills strained the emotions of the compassionate nurse. The hospital sisters worked seven days a week, although later in the 1950s that policy was changed, and they were given one day off a week. Somehow, outside the long hours working in the operating room, Sister Joachim managed to study for and finally receive a Bachelor of Science degree. But she still pursued her music. Sister Victoria Marie, one of Joachim's religious sisters who worked with her at the Pueblo hospital, recalled the 1957 ceremony that united the newly rebuilt St. Mary's Hospital with the old CDF&I Corwin hospital. Sister Mary Joachim wrote a Mass to commemorate the occasion. She practiced the voice parts of the Mass with the hospital staff, and the performance, according to Sister Victoria Marie who took part in the chorus, "was thrilling."[1] Joachim also found time to write a Christmas Mass, the themes taken from variations of Christmas carols. Later, in Santa Fe, the sisters performed her Christmas Mass at St. Vincent's.[2]

Sister Mary Joachim had been working eight years in Pueblo's St. Mary's-Corwin Hospital when the call came from the Cincinnati Sisters for her to return to Santa Fe as administrator of St Vincent Hospital. She was thirty-eight years old. She was delighted with the prospect of working again in the capital city and seeing the friends she had made in her short time there. As soon as she arrived, however, she discovered that much work lay ahead of her, work well beyond her experience as a nurse, well beyond what she could have anticipated.

As with many hospitals in the United States, the Great Depression of the 1930s and the subsequent war had taken a drastic financial toll on Santa Fe's only hospital. There had been little money available throughout the nation to replace ageing, obsolete equipment, and the city's small, 1910 hospital— although enlarged over the years from 75 to 125 beds—

was one of the oldest. As soon as the war was over, Congress passed the Hospital Survey and Construction Act of 1946—more commonly known as the Hill-Burton Act—to deal with the deterioration of the nation's hospitals. The Act was a priority on President Truman's agenda for rebuilding the nation's infrastructure that had suffered neglect during the previous two decades. During the war, the Army Medical Corps had built and operated a hospital, Burns General Hospital, on the grounds of the College of Santa Fe. The St. Vincent nurses complained that the army had taken all their specialists, leaving only eight doctors on the medical staff. After the war, the army hospital closed, and several officers who had worked in the hospital, returned to Santa Fe in a move that changed the medical community "from one that had been primarily of family physicians, to one with a preponderance of specialists."[3] A similar trend was occurring nationwide. Further, advances in medical technology meant a need for new, expensive equipment, personnel training, and expanding or replacing existing structures.

The Sisters of Charity were offered a $250,000 federal planning grant to study improvements to the old St Vincent Hospital. There was no question that the hospital had to be rescued, but the sisters were uncertain if the grant should be accepted. Santa Fe had changed after the war: the folksy parties and all-night poker games were indulgences of the past. The community's attitude toward the hospital was divided. Some of the residents believed the hospital should no longer be a Catholic institution; others wanted the sisters to remain in charge; still others wanted a new, nonsectarian general county hospital. There was much back and forth in the newspaper "Letters to the Editor"—it was the $250,000 question, proclaimed an editorial in *The Santa Fe New Mexican*.[4]

In 1949, the sisters decided to accept the grant; it was clear that a new hospital building was needed. Sister Mary Joachim was working at the hospital during the planning process, but only briefly in Santa Fe and busy with her nursing activities, she was not involved in the early planning stages. The noted local architect, John Gaw Meem, was chosen to design the new facility. The task of soliciting and coordinating the financing for the project and fund-raising in the community, as well as dealing with the building plans, fell to the then-current administrator, Sr. Ann Teresa Neary. Sister Ann also had to handle the inevitable hassles of managing the old hospital while the new one was under construction, with attendant parking problems and the need to ensure that emergency access would be always available. Some $300,000 for new equipment was raised from donations by the community, and the federal government, through Hill-Burton funds, contributed $1.2 million; the Sisters of Charity loaned almost $2 million. The groundbreaking took place in January 1951. Building a new and expanded hospital meant that the old historic buildings on the site would have to be demolished—the small hospital, built in 1886, and the little adobe that had been Archbishop Lamy's quarters. The original adobe hospital, dating from 1865 also needed to be razed, as was Seton Hall, formerly the convent and nurses residence. A year later, the orphanage was closed and razed. The old, 1910 St. Vincent Hospital where Sister Joachim had worked was renamed "Marian Hall." It became the convent for the sister-nurses and the new location of the Licensed Practical Nurse (LPN) nursing school, originally established in 1921. The three-story building also contained a kitchen for the convent, a chapel, a library, and assembly rooms.

Architect Meem's new 211-bed fireproof hospital rose on Palace Avenue in an approximation of New Mexico's historic "territorial style," and in January, two years after the ground-breaking, the new hospital was dedicated to the community by Archbishop Edwin Byrne. Thousands came to see the new facility during a two-day open house event, one of whom was Abe Silver, a local businessman, who for several nights had climbed up to a window in the old hospital to view his newborn son. The new St Vincent's was lauded in national hospital journals. One articled noted that while it was "not the largest or most magnificent, it has few to equal it in completeness."[5]

In preparation to serve the new hospital, local community leader Virginia Van Solen and several friends established the Hospital Auxiliary in 1951. Composed of community volunteers, the Auxiliary members donated thousands of hours to benefit the new St. Vincent's. The organization continues today, providing comfort to the patients and assistance to the nurses. For years the auxiliary held community fairs to raise funds for the purchase of new equipment. The members staff a gift shop and a hospital information desk, take flowers to the patients, manage a mobile library, and perform countless small tasks to keep the hospital running smoothly. Marguerite Claffey was one of the early organizers of the auxiliary; she knew the hospital well, having been one of the children who used to slide down the banisters. Claffey had become friends with Sister Mary Joachim during the period Sister was Superintendent of Nurses in the old hospital. In 1960, the administrator, Sister Mary Vivian, left after only a year and returned to Ohio, so the hospital had to find a replacement. Claffey wrote to the Sisters of Charity asking if they would send an "experienced administrator." Marguerite Claffey knew the president of the Sisters of Charity, and it is very likely she followed up her letter with a phone call requesting that Sr. Mary Joachim be chosen.[6]

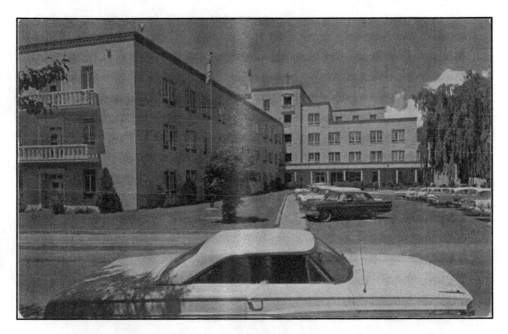

St. Vincent Hospital on Palace Avenue, opened 1953.
Photograph: New Mexico History Museum Photo Archives no. 43460.

When, in 1960, Sister Mary Joachim returned to Santa Fe in her administrative position, the hospital was in a financial crisis. The costs to cover the nonpaying indigents had escalated to fifteen per cent per year, and the general occupancy rate was only fifty percent. The hospital wasn't breaking even. Given the grim situation, the Cincinnati Sisters were unable to make payments on their $2 million loan, covering only the interest from revenues from their other hospitals and schools. No capital improvements had been made, and in the fast pace of medical innovation, the life of much of the equipment had passed. Further, although many had helped with fund-raising and service, perhaps more in the community still did not support the relatively new institution. The issues that had come up eleven years earlier during planning for the new facility were still being aired. The problems would have staggered an experienced administrator, and Sister Mary Joachim, although she had recently taken some graduate courses in hospital administration at St Louis University, had never managed a hospital before.

The first task that faced the new administrator was to try to turn around the hospital's reputation in the eyes of the community. Sister Joachim had heard the rumors: obsolete, too expensive, poor service. Some even referred to the hospital as "Saint Victim's." She decided to launch a massive public relations assault. Public relations work, which often came down to knocking on the community's doors, hobnobbing at cocktail parties with possible donors—dark rum her preference, but never to excess—and pleading before public bodies, would come hard for this spiritual nun who would much rather use what little spare time she had either listening to music or in quiet contemplation and prayer. The hospital lawyer complained it was undignified for a nun to go around town speaking in public and soliciting funds. Dignified or not, Sister Joachim knew she had no choice. She had been called, and she plunged into the project with characteristic efficacy and conviction. Later she recalled,

> I guess my lack of experience was an advantage, since I didn't really know how impossible things were. I just went to work to do what had to be done.... [T]hose first few years were so

tragic they were almost comical. Our scientific equipment needed replacement, the roof leaked, the basement flooded, and people were stuck in the elevator almost every day. If you can think of a hospital problem, we had it…. Just when it appeared impossible, some of our Santa Fe friends would come to the rescue. We existed almost on a day to day basis."[7]

Sister Joachim had long ago lost the dream of a music career. She was now a hospital administrator twenty-four hours a day. "I probably would have been a poor artist, a bad musician, and a pauper when I died," she joked to a reporter. "You never know what God has in mind."[8]

Often, Sister Joachim didn't turn off the light in her office until eleven o'clock at night. To add to her duties managing some four hundred fifty employees in fourteen departments—the city's largest source of private employment—and ensuring the hospital continued to meet the standards for accreditation, she had to soothe a sometimes ruffled medical staff, juggle a budget of millions, and try to convince the community to support her. Additionally, she was the superior of the religious sisters who worked at the hospital and at other venues in Santa Fe. The sister-nurses answered to her both as their religious boss and as their employer boss, which sometimes led to conflict. At first, relates Sister Pat Bernard who worked for Sister Mary Joachim in those early years, Joachim was progressive and fun-loving—joking with the sisters, bringing wine into the convent in the evenings, and teaching them to appreciate classical music. One of the sisters recalls that Sister Joachim taught her to understand the theory of music composition, lessons that she has valued all her life, and encouraged her to explore her artistic interests, allowing her to use the Marian Hall basement as a sculpture studio. But the pressures of the hospital's problems began to wear on the overworked nun. She became much more rigid: "If you didn't agree with her, move on," was the attitude her friend recalled.[9] And gradually they did move on. It was also the period of Vatican II, with the loosening of some of the more rigid Church traditions. Sister Joachim found this hard to take. The Cincinnati Sisters decided in the mid-'sixties that the long, black floor-length habit was no longer necessary, and should be replaced by a modest, more practical blue dress—the "Seton dress," named after the founder of the Sisters of Charity, Elizabeth Seton. The black cap would be exchanged for a simple head covering—the "veil." Until then, the sister-nurses had worn the traditional long habit and cap, except that for them, the habit was white. As a traditionalist, Sister Joachim was sad to see the change, but following her vow of obedience, as well as realizing its practicality, she did adopt the new dress. Still later, after the sisters were allowed the option to wear lay clothes, she even changed to a discrete dark business suit for her public appearances. But always wearing the veil over her hair. The sister-nurses wore the veil, too, but later changed to a standard staff nurses' uniform. Some years later, Sister Joachim wrote an indignant letter to a reviewer of the1970s TV mystery show featuring Tom Bosley as Father Dowling and Tracy Nelson as Sister Steve. According to Tracy Nelson, some nuns had told her that the only unrealistic thing about the show was that Sister Steve wore a long black habit. This raised the ire of Sister Joachim's traditionalist soul. Her angry response insisted there was nothing "unrealistic" about wearing a habit:

> There are a good many of us out here still wearing habits, and we are far from being unrealistic."… There are many sisters in habits who work among the poor, the prostitutes, the drug population, and in foreign countries, and who face the very real world the same as those who choose not to wear habits.… Would you say Mother Teresa of Calcutta and her sisters are "unrealistic"?[10]

The sister-nurses and Sister Joachim had to accommodate themselves to situations that would occur in the New Mexico hospital that were outside their past experience. In a 1964 issue of the Sisters of Charity magazine for the Order, *Unity,* Sister Joachim described the three cultures of New Mexico as blending a tradition-filled way of life. These traditions sometimes required the nurses to deal with Spanish *brujas* (witches) and Indian medicine men. "Often patients come in [to the hospital] with bags of herbs tied to their bodies 'to cure the disease and ease the pain.' Tax stamps from tobacco are stuck on cuts and bruises in the belief this will prevent infection." These incidents added to the mystery of New Mexico, a mystery that Sister Joachim responded to: "All this makes New Mexico truly the Land of Enchantment, where spirits, lifted to the turquoise skies, glorify God."[11]

Sister Joachim "ran a tight ship," one admiring friend noted. "And she really knew her numbers. The hospital was exceedingly well managed and spotlessly clean. In public, she was able to hide her worries behind an engaging smile and a wonderful sense of humor."[12] But for some it was a stressful environment: some of the regular employees and some of the sister-nurses left to find work elsewhere, some even left the Order. Starting with twenty-nine nuns when Sister Joachim first came to the hospital, over the years the number fluctuated, some leaving, new ones coming, but at the end of her stay, the number finally reduced to five, including the administrator. Of course there are many personal reasons the sisters left. Some were called to take other positions, others left the Order to marry or to take jobs outside the religious environment. Religious orders everywhere were losing members, especially after Vatican II, and the governance of the orders was becoming less focused on members' vows of "obedience" and more on encouraging personal initiative.[13] One of the nurses who later left, and who subsequently married a monk, described her decision to leave the Order as part of her "spiritual walk." Several years later, she recalled her time at the hospital with great affection:

> We were up at 5:30. First there was Morning Prayer in the convent chapel. Then Mass was at 6:15. People came to the convent for Mass from the outside, it was always open to employees and friends. Then we had breakfast in the convent and started work in the hospital at seven. We had a list of patients who wanted to take Communion. The hospital was very quiet. We would walk down the halls, ringing a little bell to announce Communion. It was very peaceful and beautiful. After work we had supper in the convent with Sister, then perhaps some entertainment before evening prayer."[14]

The New Mexico legislature passed the Indigent Hospital Claims Act, enabling New Mexico counties to be responsible for indigent care. Santa Fe County decided on a proposition that would add an indigent tax onto the property assessments to help the hospital. In 1964 the proposition was defeated, four to one. Sister Mary Joachim faced the possibility that Saint Vincent Hospital would close.

By 1965, the situation was drastic. The Sisters of Charity had been operating Santa Fe's only hospital for a hundred years, and the problems, although most of a different order from those of a hundred years earlier, were in some ways the same. The indigent care bills were crushing. The hospital equipment was becoming obsolete, and the annual budget deficit was near $350,000. Payroll after payroll had to be heavily subsidized by the Sisters of Charity, and they still had made no payments on the 1951 loan. Between 1960 and 1963, the Cincinnati Sisters poured over three million dollars into free charity care at St. Vincent's. Things were so dire that Archbishop James P. Davis sold his emerald and diamond episcopal ring to help pay for hospital equipment. Greer Garson came to town to help raise funds, and the Lensic Theatre showed the film, *The Singing Nun*, which featured Garson in the role of the Mother Prioress. Mayor Pat Hollis proclaimed "Greer Garson Day" in Santa Fe. The eighth graders of the Cristo Rey Civics Club sent out a thousand letters, painted 200 posters, and set out collection cans. They wrote to politicians and professional athletes; Mickey Mantle's manager responded and endorsed the club's project, as did US Representative Johnny Walker from Washington, and Governor Jack Campbell. All of this helped, but much more was needed. "I don't mean to imply the entire picture was dark," Sister Joachim commented in a statement to the Sisters of Charity. "There were some wonderful experiences, and I was making friends whom I will treasure the rest of my life."[15] Yet even with the hospital in terrible financial shape, Sister Joachim, presented a confident attitude to the public. One wouldn't know she was contemplating the possible closure of the institution. One *New Mexican* reporter noted:

When you meet Sister you immediately feel her warmth and interest in people and their problems. When you talk to her she makes you feel your problem is the most important one in the world and you relax because you know she will come up with the right solution. Her faith and common sense, her genuine desire to help people in all walks of life flow out to everyone she meets. Her smile envelops you in understanding and sympathy.[16]

Sister Joachim was acknowledged widely by hospital and civic organizations for her efforts to turn around the situation. An article in *The New Mexican* reported that the hospital administrator "rivals the nation's top business women."[17] Another article stated: "Sister possesses business capabilities that often go unnoticed in a man, but sparkle brightly in this age when recognition of executive ability in women is being stressed in all levels of endeavor."[18] In 1966, she was elected president of the New Mexico Hospital Association's Board of Trustees, was a fellow of the American College of Hospital Administrators, and was twice elected as delegate at large to the American Hospital Association from Region 8, covering Colorado, Utah, Idaho, Arizona as well as New Mexico. She organized and was first president of the New Mexico Northern Area Hospital Council. For several years she was a member of the New Mexico Blue Cross board, and in Washington DC, she was appointed to the national Health Education and Welfare Committee for Migrant Health. In this position Sister spent time over the next six years visiting migrant labor camps. Concerned about problems of drug abuse, she became a board member of La Puerta, a local abuse program. The governor of New Mexico conferred on her the title of Colonel, Aide-de-Camp. Fortunately, it was only an honorary title, since theoretically it required that she follow the "usage and discipline of the United States Army." One honor she received that especially pleased her, given the contentious attitude toward the hospital by some in the community, was her selection by the local Jaycees as "1966 Boss of the Year."

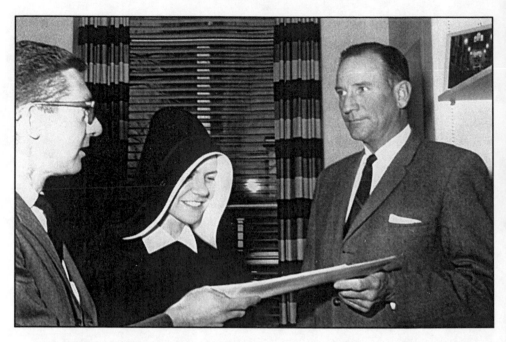

Sister Mary Joachim receives an award from Dr. Bergere Kenney (left) and Ed Brosseau. Photograph: David Kenney collection.

"I've been criticized for going to so many meetings," Sister commented to a reporter from *The New Mexican,* "but you have to go. At these outside meetings you share ideas, you learn about new health care concepts and cutting costs." She went on to say that the hardest thing about her job was the decision-making. "As President Truman said, 'the buck stops here.' You don't make decisions without input, but the time comes for one person to make the final decision....You've got to have discipline and rules in a hospital because you're dealing with human life. If people are not responsible, from the man who cleans the floor through the medical staff, lives are at stake."

The reporter suggested Sister might consider her position a symbolic victory for the women's liberation movement. Joachim responded, "I have not thought of my job in that way. I do it because that's what I'm supposed to do." As for women's lib: "What do they want to be liberated from—their womanhood?" She noted, however, that she was well aware that women face discrimination, but that she herself had never felt discriminated against in the medical field; "perhaps," she suggested, "because the medical profession is accustomed to seeing sisters in the administrative role in the many Catholic hospitals throughout the country." She confessed she never had any ambition to become a hospital administrator: "I was a happy nurse...because it was a wonderful thing to give service in that way." But when the call came to take over the administration of St. Vincent's, she said she just did the job she was given to the best of her ability.[19] As in most hospitals, there were occasional problems with the physicians. One doctor recalled that in dealing with the medical staff, Sister Joachim was "tough":

> She had to be. She kicked out some doctors who were "tanked." And one for having an affair with one of the staff. Some in the town didn't like the hospital because it was Catholic. Some in the community as well as some of the doctors wanted the hospital to perform abortions, but Sister Joaquin wouldn't allow it. There were always problems with the Catholics versus the non-Catholics. And some of the doctors were incompetent. One claimed his records were lost in the war. I don't think he was really a doctor. And some doctors treated the nurses with disrespect. One doctor, who botched an operation, had told the nurse to get out of the operating room, then tried to blame her for his mistake."[20]

Sister Joachim had a plan. She determined the Sisters of Charity should relinquish control of the hospital and turn it over to a community board of directors. With the hospital finances a losing proposition, it seemed the only thing to do would be to let the community be responsible for it's survival. For the Cincinnati Sisters, this was a revolutionary idea. They indeed had sold other of their hospitals before, but certainly not simply turned one over to a nonprofit group of community leaders. They agreed to consider the suggestion.

Before such a step could be taken, however, something had to be done about the charity problem. With the help of State Senator Alex Martinez and Representative Bruce King, who at the time was Speaker of the House, Sister Joachim lobbied a bill through the legislature that allowed a county to propose a sales tax to pay for indigent hospital expenses. "Perhaps the [earlier] choice of a property owner's assessment was both unfortunate and unfair," Sister reflected later, "but we had to start somewhere."[21] She went to the County Board of Commissioners, explaining that since a property tax assessment was unacceptable to the voters, they should use the new law to propose a percentage on the sales tax. One quarter of one percent would perhaps be acceptable to the voters, she determined, an amount so small to individual consumers they wouldn't even notice it on the sales slip. Carlos Martinez, a newly elected County Commissioner, championed the idea. "It was the best thing I was ever involved in," he recalled years later. And lauding Sister Mary Joachim for her service, Martinez recounted, "She was like a living saint to me. When you talked to her, you knew she was close to the Lord."[22] *The New Mexican* supported the sales tax idea with articles and editorials. Sister Joachim, accompanied by her friend, Marguerite Claffey, went door-to-door all over the city and county, explaining the hospital's desperate circumstances and urging people to vote for the sales tax. She spoke at community meetings, at churches, at the Chamber of Commerce, at the City Council. This time she was successful. In April 1968, the sales tax passed in a four-to-one reverse of the earlier vote. It was a rousing vote of confidence from the community. When the money started to come in, the hospital gradually surfaced from under its load of unpaid bills.

Later, Sister Joachim could look back and laugh.

> One thing about reaching bottom, there is only one way to go— up. And from that time things started to improve for us. The people of Santa Fe began to recognize the problems we faced, and slowly we were to receive assistance from a larger segment of the community. I really think 1965 was the turning point for the hospital.[23]

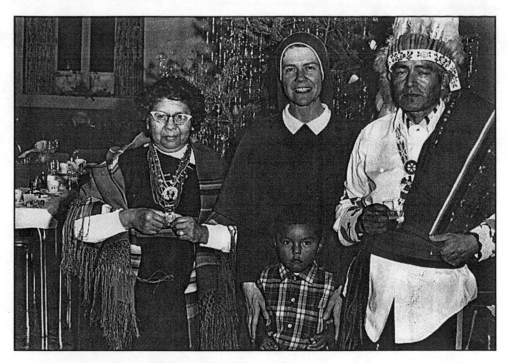

The Trujillos of San Juan Pueblo receive the hospital's ten-year service pins.
Photograph: Sisters of Charity Archives.

In the 1972 hospital newsletter, Mary Joaquin recalled her discouragement of the previous years:

> There was no support here for the hospital. I could not see the Sisters of Charity continuing to pour money into the institution. It was ridiculous to go back each year to the City and beg for $25,000, which lasted half a year. So I told the Sisters of Charity to let us sink or swim.[24]

An intensive fund drive in the community, sponsored by the Hospital Auxiliary, had raised $250,000 in tax-exempt donations to replace some of the obsolete and worn out equipment, and in 1966, Medicare and Medicaid payments became available. By the next year, Sister Joachim believed that with the charity problem under control, if not completely solved, she could concentrate on her plan to turn the hospital over to the community. It was a plan, she said later, "to phase myself out."[25] In 1967, Sister Joachim took a group of Santa Fe citizens to the Ohio Motherhouse. The group requested the governing board of the Sisters of Charity to allow a local board of trustees to be formed, and to plan a program for turnover of the assets to the new board in the next few years so that expansion or replacement of the hospital could be realized. At that time, the Cincinnati Sisters were in the process of upgrading their St Joseph Hospital in Albuquerque; they couldn't afford the needed expansion of St Vincent's. Their main concern was that a new community board retire their 26-year old debt, and this was uppermost for Sister Joachim as she planned the community "takeover."

Despite the stress of financial problems over the years, people who knew Sister Joachim well commented on her wit, her wonderful warm smile, and her tolerance for the more unseemly of some of the doctors' antics. One doctor, a psychiatrist, recounted his first meeting with Sister.

"I was a newcomer in Santa Fe. I had opened my own office, but I had no relation to the medical staff of the hospital. One evening I was invited to a party at the home of one of the head doctors at the hospital. Suddenly, a call came in that there was a psychiatric emergency at the hospital—a man was hysteric and was having a seizure. One of the guests, Dr. Chris Mengis, turned to me and said 'Well, you're the only psychiatrist here. You'd better get over there.' Dr. Mengis, who was famous for his red Rolls Royce and who moonlighted as a member of the volunteer fire department, was also famous as a jokester, but at the time, I didn't know this. I went immediately to the hospital and took care of the patient. No one at the hospital knew who I was. A few days later I got a call from Sister Joachim, asking me to come to her office. 'I understand you helped one of our patients the other night,' she said with her characteristic broad smile. 'I guess you didn't realize it, but you passed Chris's test.' Her eyes were twinkling, and I realized I had been set up. Since I was a newcomer, they wanted to test me to see if I could deal with the situation. Sister Joachim invited me to join her staff."[26]

3

∼†∼

For years New Mexico had had a problem attracting physicians because the legislature didn't allow reciprocity of licenses issued by other states. A doctor wishing to be licensed in New Mexico had to repeat an examination in what were essentially the basic science classes he or she had taken in the first two years of medical school. The requirement was a deterrent, and in 1968 a bill was pending in the legislature to allow reciprocity. One day while Sister Joachim was having a conversation with a visiting doctor in the hallway of the hospital, the assistant administrator, George Boal, arrived in the hall carrying a sign saying, "The bill passed!" The visitor asked what the sign meant. Before she could answer, a woman doctor walked up and announced: "It means free beer for everyone!" Sister Joaquin had to take a lot from this woman, an orthopedic surgeon who was notorious, among other scandalous activities, for playing tennis topless at the racquet club. Sister was relieved that at least the doctor didn't walk around the hospital thus unattired.

One friend, who let slip some rather foul language while talking to the nun, apologized for his indiscretion. Sister Joachim laughed, and said, "You don't even come close to the cussing of the orthopedic surgeons. I've heard everything!"[1] Apparently Sister felt the orthopedists were the worst of the lot. Years later, she inadvertently came upon an anti-AIDS poster on the desk of a doctor friend. The poster portrayed a humorously vulgar picture of two men locked in coitus. The doctor apologized that she had seen it, but Sister Joaquin merely responded with a smile that she might have known it would be on the desk of an orthopedic surgeon.

Under Sister Joachim's leadership, the hospital was able to make substantial improvements. A new coronary care unit was added, the first in the state, and the cardiology lab was remodeled and named for Will Harrison, who, as editor of *The New Mexican*, had made the newspaper a great supporter. An intensive care unit and a respiratory therapy unit were opened, and subsequently a nuclear medicine unit. The only two psychiatrists on staff, however, couldn't agree on establishing a psychiatric unit. One supported shock therapy; the other was determinedly against such treatment. So the hospital went without a psychiatric unit, until years later when the Behavioral Science Center opened in 1985.[2] It was important to keep upgrading the hospital equipment, even when the hospital was so overcrowded that clearly it soon had to be expanded or rebuilt at another location. With beds in the halls and in the alcoves, the Fire Department was extremely unhappy with the administration; patients, visitors, and police crowded into the ER, long lines of patients waited for their X-rays. Planning standards required two and a half parking spaces per hospital bed. The number of beds was by now reduced to 201, with 232 total spaces to serve visitors, a hundred doctors, and five hundred employees. At peak hours, on-site parking was nonexistent.

In 1968, Sister Mary Joachim celebrated her Silver Jubilee as a Sister of Charity. The event was held in Marian Hall with an Agape Mass—a Mass of generosity to the poor. Archbishop Davis conducted the Mass, and Joachim renewed her vows to the Order. The service was followed by an elegant buffet dinner hosted by the Hospital Auxiliary, the hall adorned with decorations of silver and turquoise. A proud Aunt Nelle, the woman who had started young Gina Bitler on her nursing career, came from Ohio to attend the ceremony.

Also in 1968 Sister Joachim took the first steps to implement her plan to turn the hospital over to the community, a plan she had been working out for the last six years. The hospital had had a lay citizen advisory board for several years, but, as the Santa Fe visitors had explained to the governing board of the sisters in Ohio, Sister Joachim's plan was to create a new board of trustees that would actually be in charge of policy. The proposed board would ultimately take ownership of the hospital, and decide what should to be done to resolve the need for expansion.

The hospital staff put notices in the newspapers advertising for trustees for the volunteer board, and the advisory board members contacted community groups. Only a few responded, and the first Board of Trustees consisted of thirteen members: seven from the community, five Sisters of Charity from the nursing staff, and Sister Mary Joaquin. The board was formed "rather by parthenogenesis" in the words of Dr. Bergere Kenney, the first chairman. Dr. Kenney was chief of the medical staff at St. Vincent's and a professor of medicine at the University of New Mexico.

The hospital, although still owned by the Cincinnati Order, became legally St. Vincent Hospital, Inc., a nondenominational, nonprofit corporation. At the request of the new board, an important part of the agreement with the Sisters of Charity was that the sisters would remain at work in the hospital, at least until ownership was legally transferred. "Modesty probably prevents Sr. Mary Joachim and Assistant Administrator George Boal from pointing out that it was really their idea," Dr. Kenney told a reporter.[3] The Cincinnati sisters would no longer set policy. The board members would serve without pay, and would be responsible for all management and operational policies of the hospital, except for physician standards, which were determined by the medical staff. Daily operations would continue under Sister Mary Joachim.

Sister Joaquin realized that the people of Santa Fe would be more willing to support St. Vincent's as a community corporation than as a Catholic hospital, and although the changeover was what she had worked for, she also had concerns:

> God help us if it ever becomes less than a Christian hospital. The thing that makes us different from other hospitals is our commitment to the whole person. To us, it's a little more than just putting bones back together."[4]

Although owned by a Catholic Order, the hospital encouraged leaders of all faiths to work with the doctors and patients in the recuperation process of the whole being—spiritually as well as physically. "Our goal," Joachim said, "is to recognize the dignity of man through total patient-centered care."[5] Nevertheless, as the administrator of a Catholic hospital, Sister Joachim followed the edicts of the Church regarding the sanctity of life and birth control. She reports, in an informational letter addressed to the Sisters of Charity as a group, that she was continually "harassed by those favoring certain changes in ethical procedures contrary to the teachings of the Catholic Church."[6] Which didn't mean that on the birth control issue, she wasn't averse to "looking the other way" in certain cases. One woman, having just given birth in the hospital to her fourth child, told Sister that she didn't want more children, and asked to be allowed to have a tubal ligation. Sister refused her, but then later, rather surreptitiously, suggested that one of the doctors could perform the procedure for her in Española.

Sister Jane was a Sister of Charity social worker at St. Vincent's. Sister Joachim had asked her to come out from Ohio and help her with the practical and social needs of the patients. Sister Jane spoke Spanish, having worked for years as a teacher in Peru. Her work in Santa Fe was to follow up on the elderly patients after they left the hospital. Jane would make the rounds of the neighborhoods, doing little tasks to help out. Once she helped a woman hang out her laundry; for another, she cleaned the house. She drove people to doctors' appointments, took them grocery shopping, cooked meals for them, or perhaps just visited with them. "Some of the people were very wealthy," Sister Jane said. "They just wanted someone to talk to. Some of the doctors' wives helped, too. You made a lot of friends in Santa Fe that way." One of the elderly Hispanic men she visited was a paraplegic, confined all day to a wheelchair. "I asked him to tell me his history—and oh my lands! He started this recitation … and he just went on and on, and was waving his arms about. We had the nicest time."[7]

Sister Jane told a story that well describes how the philosophy of the hospital under Sister Mary Joachim's direction was "a little more than just putting bones back together":

A Mexican national was brought in. He'd been in a terrible accident in a lumberyard where he worked, and his leg was broken in several places. After the surgery, I went to talk to him. He assured me that his *patron* would be coming. "He has my money, four hundred dollars. That's my salary. I know he will come." I doubted we would ever see that *patron,* but I alerted the staff to watch for him and to call me if he came. Well, surprisingly, the *patron* did come, and I asked him if he had brought the man's money. "Yes, but it's out in my truck." I was pretty sure the man would just drive away, so I went with him to his truck, and made him give me the four hundred dollars. We were told that the INS was coming to get our patient and take him back to Mexico, and we knew that they wouldn't let him leave the country with more than forty dollars in his pocket. So the nurses opened their patient's cast and put his money inside and bandaged him up again, leaving out forty dollars. The INS agent asked us if he had any money, and I said, "Yes, he has forty dollars in his back pocket." The agent said that was OK, and the orderlies carried him out to the INS van on a stretcher.[8]

4

~†~

*T*he first task of the new Board of Trustees was to take a crash course in hospital management and administration of a $3 million budget, $2 million of which was payroll. The next was to address the much-needed expansion of the facility. Daily, some seven hundred people—employees and patients—occupied the hospital, and by this time the facility had become seriously overcrowded, with beds lining the hallways. Space was also made for the overload in some of the empty rooms in the adjacent Marian Hall. A group of physicians and community leaders formed the Key Club, whose initial project was to raise funds to hire a consulting firm to determine the best way to address the hospital expansion. A Malibu firm, Medical Planning Association, was chosen. The consultants determined there were three options possible: expand the existing hospital with a two-story addition; build an entirely new hospital in another location; or construct a new satellite facility away from downtown, retaining the existing hospital.[1]

The consideration of the options created another maelstrom of controversy in the community. The board quickly determined the first option was much too expensive. There wasn't enough room to add onto the existing structure and provide adequate parking without having to purchase high cost land immediately to the south. The Historical Site Board had set a height limit of sixty-five feet in the area, and the hospital was already at sixty-five feet. Nevertheless, the first option—expanding the existing hospital— was preferred by many of the doctors, who didn't want to leave the downtown area where they had established their offices in proximity to the hospital. But traffic had increased considerably in the area since the hospital was built and was negatively impacting nearby residences. Further, improvements to Paseo de Peralta would cut off frontage, putting patient rooms right at the street. Both cost and traffic were reasons to reject the third—the satellite option—as well.

Despite the many voices against moving the hospital, it seemed logical to the committee to choose the second option—building an entirely new hospital in another location. The region had grown in the last years and growth was expected to continue. A large hospital with adequate parking on a site that would provide opportunity for future expansion seemed to many, if not all, the proper solution. It was the solution favored by Sister Mary Joaquin and the other members of the Board of Trustees. Hence, regardless of the disagreements in the community, the Board of Trustees began the search for a site to move the hospital. After reviewing fourteen different locations, they purchased a forty-three acre site on St. Michaels Drive south of the downtown for $215,600 with a $20,000 down payment from an anonymous friend. A master planning committee, headed by Dr. Richard Streeper, set about working with architects Elias Kaplan of San Francisco and Philippe Register of Santa Fe. The committee members held meetings with state, county, and local health officials; surveys were compiled of the present building and projected needs; requirements of every department were reviewed. Suggestions were solicited from the doctors and nurses, administrative and other staff. The committee soon had drawn up a conceptual plan; it listed anticipated future requirements, and was discussed and argued about in public meetings for the next six years.

The indigent fund, along with some financial help from the city and county and from community fundraising, had allowed the Board of Trustees to begin making some payments on the Sisters of Charity's 2 million dollar loan, and the sisters agreed to turn over ownership when half the debt was paid. But the charity write-offs were still costing the hospital between \$100,000 to \$300,000 a year, an amount that had to be made up by local government help, community fundraisers, and hospital charges. Along with Santa Fe County, only Rio Arriba County imposed the quarter-cent tax, but St. Vincent's was still required to take in everyone, regardless of their ability to pay—the Sisters of Charity insisted on that. "We're glad to serve here," Sister Joachim stated to a reporter, "but we can only give a certain percentage of free services before our back is cracked."[2]

A primary concern of Sister Joaquin was for St. Vincent's, despite the hospital's financial woes, to be able to maintain a high quality of service. An interesting twist on "quality of service" is another Sister Jane story:

A man was brought in one night in terrible shape from an accident. The nurses put a trach in him, so he couldn't speak, and he was on a respirator. We knew nothing about him. Three days later a woman appeared at the hospital door in the middle of the night. 'I am the wife of Francisco,' she said. I took her up to our patient's room. When she saw her husband with all the tubes and oxygen and the respirator, she was beside herself. Two of the nurses' aides took the woman home with them and gave her a bed and food. We kept Francisco at the hospital for a month, but the situation was hopeless, and we were just keeping him alive with machines. We finally had to tell her that we had to pull the plug. She took the news bravely, but insisted that she must take his body back to Mexico. "I'll never be able to see his grave," she wailed. We called the undertaker, who said that it would cost \$2000 to send the body across the border in the required hermetically sealed coffin. The hospital couldn't afford that. "If you could get the body down to the Rio, to the bridge," the wife said, "a man will meet us with an ambulance and take him across." We found a small prop plane, and she and I flew with the body wrapped in a sheet. She was terrified; the little plane flew so close to the ground, and she'd never been in a plane before. Sure enough, there was a man there to take the body across. It cost us, but I'm so glad we could do it for her.[3]

About this time, Sister Mary Joachim decided to change her name from "Joachim" to "Joaquin." The reason, she said, was that Joachim was hard for her friends to pronounce. "Perhaps," said a friend, laughing. "But it may also be because the governor insisted on calling her 'Sister Yokum.'"[4] According to board member Abe Silver, some of the board members had given up on her name altogether, and called her simply "Mary Jo."

The Board of Trustee's challenge for building a new hospital on St. Michael's Drive was finding the estimated $12 - $13 million for construction and another $4 million or more for equipment. And the Sisters of Charity's debt was still outstanding. To make matters worse, in 1973, the country was in the midst of an energy crisis, and St. Vincent's was in for belt-tightening. The board instituted a voluntary staff leave of one day a month. There were no lay-offs, but overtime was restricted, and to save energy, lights were turned off in the halls and water and gas were conserved.

Federal wage-price controls restricted hospitals from raising prices, but not those of the suppliers. And Sister Mary Joaquin was frustrated by other federal rules: Medicare required shorter hospital stays, and federal bureaucrats made the decisions on patient dismissals. This often conflicted with what she felt were a patient's needs. An additional problem was the lack of nursing homes in the Santa Fe area. Joaquin was deeply concerned about patients whose continued hospitalization could not be justified under Medicare regulations, but required post-hospitalization in nursing homes.

The proposed new hospital was partly dependent on a community fund drive, the board hoping for at least $2 million from the drive and another $2 million from the anticipated sale of the existing building once it was vacated. Fortunately, the hospital was able to transfer financial responsibility for the practical nursing school to the vocational school in El Rito, the state education department providing the funding.[5] But the emergency room, serving 16,000 patients a year, needed 24-hour

hour medical staff coverage at a cost of $111,000. The City dipped into its revenue-sharing funds for $12,000 to help the situation. Then in March 1973, the state Advisory Hospital Council declared the existing facility nonconforming because of obsolescence. This declaration would jeopardize any possible federal assistance, forcing the City of Santa Fe to foot the cost of any expansion or remodeling at the present site.

For some time, Sister Joaquin had realized that she needed a graduate degree in hospital administration. She had taken some graduate courses in administration earlier in her career, but had not finished the curriculum for a degree. In her position as CEO, her lack of advanced credentials had caused the hospital to loose three grants in the previous four years, as well as causing her to be turned down for certain speaking engagements. She found a course leading to a master's degree at University of Notre Dame, and the Sisters of Charity were willing to pay her tuition. The courses were taught over the summer, and required three summers to fulfill the requirements. With the ongoing planning and financial strategizing for the new hospital and her administrative duties managing the present hospital, it was, of course, extremely difficult for her to get away from work an entire summer. She managed to convince the university that some of the work could be done in Santa Fe, and was able to cram three summers of work into two. She wrote a thesis on setting up a community-owned, nonprofit hospital corporation, a project with which she was certainly familiar. A letter from the graduate department acknowledges that she had satisfactorily completed the requirements on her own rushed time schedule, and granted her the degree of Master of Industrial Administration in 1973.[6]

The Board of Trustees managed to raise enough money to get four local banks to hold the Sisters of Charity debt. This allowed the Cincinnati Sisters to finally transfer full ownership of the hospital to the community board in December 1973, and await the sale of the Palace Avenue hospital to receive the full payment. "As we went along," Dr. Kenney stated in a hospital newsletter, "it became obvious that if we were going to run the hospital, we had to own it." And by this time it was clear that most in the community wanted a nondenominational hospital. "The sisters were very encouraging—and they were really generous on terms."[7] Sister Mary Assunta Stang, president of the Sisters of Charity stated, "we are not selling the hospital per se, rather the Board of Trustees is taking over the remaining debt. We are really giving it as a gift to Santa Fe." Indeed, the sisters had turned over the facility—its appraised value $8 million at the time of the transfer—for only the cost of their 1951 loan.[8] The federal Department of Health, Education and Welfare promised a grant of $90,793 and a low-interest loan of $2,221,500 for the new facility. The trustees were delighted, but their enthusiasm was short-lived: President Gerald Ford threatened to put a hold on the funds.

By this time, the Board of Trustees had become more community-based, numbering twenty-two members, six of whom were sisters—of the nine still working at the hospital. Laughlin Barker, the new board president, approached Mayor Joe Valdes, requesting the City issue $12 million in industrial revenue bonds. Sister Joaquin and her assistants had lobbied the state to get legislation changed to allow local revenue bonds to be issued for health facilities. Bonds issued by the City would carry a lower interest rate than bonds issued by the hospital itself, allowing a savings of $3 million over twenty years. The City Council wanted to study the issue. Sister Joaquin pleaded with the councilors to take action immediately, and Barker urged them not to "impede" the new hospital.

Some in the audience questioned if the new hospital really needed so much money; others were concerned that the debt would mean a rise in hospital rates; still others questioned if a new hospital was needed at all. The council was concerned whether the City would be responsible if the hospital defaulted on the bonds. The hospital attorney, Seth Montgomery, assured the members the City was not liable. Dr. Edward Goodrich told the council that a majority of the physicians in two polls over the last three years opposed the move; Attorney Montgomery countered that a majority did indeed support the move. To settle the argument, a new poll of seventy doctors on the medical staff was quickly taken: 41 in favor, 23 against, 6 undecided. At the next city council meeting, the hospital people were present in force—doctors, lawyers, trustees, architects, and Sister Joaquin. There were still some in the council chamber questioning the need for a new hospital, but finally, after much heated discussion back and forth, the council voted in favor of issuing the bonds: six to one. A few weeks later, the Board of Realtors proclaimed Sister Mary Joaquin "Citizen of the Year."

5

~†~

In 1974, while the arguments continued in the community over what form the future St Vincent's should take, trouble was erupting at the hospital. The administration was faced with new and unexpected demands from the nursing staff. It was an upheaval that quickly turned ugly, both for the nurses and for the administration. Charges and countercharges flew back and forth between the two groups. Recent changes to the Taft-Hartley Act gave federal sanction to collective bargaining in nonprofit hospitals, and a group of St. Vincent nurses determined to form a union, the PPA—Professional Performance Association—to be affiliated with the New Mexico Nurses Association. The administration as well as the Board of Trustees were dead-set against it, although they claimed publicly not to be anti-union. They realized that if the nurses formed a union, they would have to bargain with it, and they were not willing to give up their authority. "Until that time," said Sister Joaquin, "I will have to deal with *all* the employees."[1]

"Salary was not a primary reason," Delma Delora, head of the nurses' group recounted later, "it was whether or not we could deliver the kind of care we were prepared to deliver with so few nurses in the hospital."[2] The nurses claimed to be suffering from fatigue, of being forced to serve too many hours of overtime, especially in the emergency room. They complained that there weren't enough RNs, and that the LPNs were doing most of the work. The administration countered that it didn't have the funds to hire more nurses. Economics determined the number of employees, and added costs would increase patient payments. Besides, the administration said it was having trouble recruiting nurses because of the confusion of the situation.

In addition to these concerns, the nurses were furious at the treatment they received from some of the doctors. At the time, it was standard practice that when a doctor entered a meeting room, a nurse had to stand up as a show of respect, and even give up her seat to him if there were no empty seats available. The nurses wanted a representative voice in running the hospital and to discuss policies on an equal basis with the administration. They protested the firing of one of their own, and 120 nurses signed the complaint. Another fired nurse told a reporter that his termination was because of disputes with several doctors, saying they treated him "like a dog."[3]

Sister Mary Joaquin was adamant that she would not give up the administration's management authority to determine the hiring and firing of staff. The nurses claimed intimidation; the administration said there was no such thing. The lawyer for the nurses, Morton Simon, claimed that administration members were harassing the leaders of the nurses' group; Owen Lopez, the hospital attorney working for Seth Montgomery's firm, said that such claims were unfounded. Lopez said that the hospital's charges were based on illegal supervisory involvement by the nurses. Such involvement is inherently coercive because of the supervisors' power to discharge and discipline those under them. "If this were a large industrial plant instead of a nonprofit hospital," Lopez said, "the supervisors would all be fired."[4]

Sister Joaquin said the PPA was using "false tactics" to make employees feel threatened and insecure, making it difficult to recruit new staff. *The New Mexican* reported that the PPA claimed the hospital administration "attempted to interrogate, coerce...and threaten to discharge several head nurses." Sister Joaquin responded: "nobody is getting fired, nobody is threatened."[5] The PPA charged its meeting notices and newsletters placed at nursing stations were removed by the administration, some within fifteen minutes of their distribution. Sister Joaquin countered, "They can peddle anything they want off-premises, but the hospital has the right to remove anything union or pro-union on hospital grounds."[6] The nurses filed a complaint against the administration with the National Labor Relations Board; the hospital filed its own unfair labor practices with the NRLB, claiming the nurses were deliberately spreading misinformation.

While the nurses and the administrative staff were facing off with their arguments, Sister Joaquin was just trying to keep things together until there would be a new hospital. She wrote in June to Sister Mary Assunta, president of the Sisters of Charity:

> I must confess the strain of trying to meet our expenses just on goods and supplies, to say nothing of salaries, is getting to me....I have been working every spare moment I can find to solicit funds. In the meantime, this place is showing its strain, wear and tear, more and more. The suction in the Operating Room went out on us last Tuesday right in the middle of the day's schedule. In having Bridgers and Paxton check it, they found we are using triple over its load capacity. Of course with the coming of two chest surgeons, and two vascular surgeons, and the addition of suction in our enlarged Recovery Room, we have just overloaded it like everything else. We've ordered two new units, with delivery in 18 weeks, at a minimum. Each day that passes offers us another challenge in trying to keep this place together safely, for at least another 2-3 years."[7]

In November 1974, the nurses' group petitioned the NLRB for an election to establish a collective bargaining unit. The sister-nurses didn't want to be involved, but they were few by this time. Sister Joaquin's view was that unions were a "haven of mediocrity." She still feared a strike and a demand for increased salaries the hospital couldn't afford. The nurses reiterated they weren't contemplating a strike, and again that salaries were not the issue. The NRLB said that if 50%-plus-one voted in favor of the proposed PPA, the union would be formed. In that case, the union would represent *all* the nurses, whether they were union members or not.

The nurses went forward with their election. All 160 RNs and LPNs were eligible to vote. The administration lost: 89% of the nurses voted to form a union. The PPA lawyer announced that collective bargaining could begin in thirty days. Dr. Goodrich, the leader of those doctors who continued to oppose the new hospital, introduced a resolution of no confidence in the administration. A vote of the medical staff defeated the resolution, 33-25. Commenting on the vote, some physicians noted that federal control of medical practice was increasingly forcing the administration to follow government rules, causing antagonism among many of them. This was indeed a narrow vote in favor of the administration. For all of her dedication to the health needs of the people of Santa Fe, Sister Joaquin had her enemies, both inside and outside the hospital.[8]

A year and a half later, the New Mexico Nurses Association, which had sponsored the new union, complained that the PPA was unprofessional and discourteous. The PPA promptly voted to end its affiliation with the association. The union continues still today as an independent bargaining unit, negotiating the salaries and working conditions for all the RN and LPN nursing staff, whether or not all are members.

The turmoil in the hospital ranks was certainly not conducive to garnering community support for the new hospital; some were still arguing over whether the hospital was even needed. Regardless of the infighting and arguments within the community, the Board of Trustees went ahead in September 1974 with plans for the groundbreaking on their site on St. Michael's Drive. They were in a rush to start the project. President Ford was still considering withholding the federal funds, and the board needed to initiate payment of the $60,000 in grading expenses to show that the new hospital was a work-in-progress. Some of the employees' children cleaned up the St Michael's site, and at the groundbreaking, the children were the first to dig their ceremonial spades into the earth, symbolic that the new hospital was being built for them, the future residents of the city. Fifteen hundred people were invited, and all the appropriate city, county and state dignitaries, along with the local clergy were present; a mariachi band played, and a hot air balloon hovered overhead.

By December, the grading machines were on site. There was an inordinate amount of grading necessary because of city height restrictions. The only way to keep the hospital within the height limit was to create below ground levels. To beat the possible funding cut-off, the grading began before the industrial revenue bonds were officially signed. Dr. Goodrich and his group of doctors and community supporters were still arguing against the project at various city venues, causing one of their colleagues on the medical staff to describe the dissenting doctors as "roaches."[9]

That Christmas, 1974, along with the relief she felt that the first steps to building the new hospital were underway, Sister Joaquin received a special present. A man who had been unable to pay his hospital bill to the Sisters of Charity at the old Marian Hall hospital thirty-nine years earlier, appeared in her office. He told the nun how grateful he was to the Sisters of Charity and that he had come to pay the $112 still owed. He paid his bill and then gave Joaquin a check for $3000 for the building fund.

In addition to clearing the ground for the new St. Vincent Hospital, the year 1975 was also an important one for Sisters of Charity everywhere. Canonized that September in Rome, the founder of the Sisters' Order, Elizabeth Ann Seton, became Saint Elizabeth Ann Seton, the first native-born American to be canonized by the Catholic Church. Sister Alice Regina, a sister-nurse at the hospital, went to Rome for the celebration. Mary Joaquin and her Sisters of Charity in Santa Fe celebrated a special Mass commemorating the event.

The bond closing took place in New York. The players were Laughlin Barker, chairman of the Board of Trustees, Attorney Seth Montgomery, Mayor Joe Valdes of Santa Fe, and agents from the investment firm of White and Weld. The funds from the A-rated bonds would be held by the Albuquerque National Bank, the construction trustee for the project. When the signing formalities were over, the group held a celebration dinner at the 21 Club. "After dinner," wrote Seth Montgomery, "we had a good round of many toasts to everyone who had played a role in the whole project; but no one was toasted more often and more enthusiastically than Sister Mary Joaquin, who had really accomplished it all." But Sister Joaquin wasn't there; the intrepid nun was afraid of flying.[10]

On September 28, 1975, construction was finally underway after being held up at the initial bid opening, the first bids having come in too high. The shell of the building slowly began to rise to the prescribed height, with an estimated completion date of mid-1977. The next June, the Board of Trustees decided to hold a "topping out" ceremony—a term that stems from barn-raisings in Northern Europe, where a tree is placed on the roof of the barn's still-unfinished structure as a good omen. The doctors and staff and board members were on the hospital roof at 7:30 in the morning. One of the doctors, who was paralyzed, had to be carried up the three flights of stairs in her wheelchair, since the elevators were not yet functioning. The group placed an evergreen tree on the roof to bring the construction good luck, to remain until the building was completed. The Board of Trustees placed a time capsule in one of the walls; they put in messages and trinkets, some put in crucifixes, one put in a mezuzah.[11] Workers found a stone that had been propped against a wall at the Palace Avenue hospital for years. Turning it over, they discovered the stone had the words "St. Vincent Hospital" carved into it. Checking old photos, it was found that the stone had once arched over the entrance to the old red brick hospital that was torn down to construct the 1953 Palace Avenue facility. The old stone sign now sits at the entrance to the new hospital.

With the hospital construction moving ahead on schedule, Sister Mary Joaquin knew that it was time for her to resign. She gave the Board of Trustees eight months notice: she and the remaining four Sisters of Charity nurses would leave at the end of November, 1976. That winter the trustees had rewritten their bylaws, and had designated a new position on the board: President of the St. Vincent Hospital Corporation. Despite Sister Joaquin's anticipated departure, the members unanimously elected her to the new position. She selected her associate, George Boal, to succeed her temporarily as administrator, and to assist the board in finding her replacement and help orient the new president to the job.

The trustees were shocked to realize that a new administrator would have to be *paid*! Sister Joaquin had been working for the last sixteen years with a minimal entry in the budget for her own salary. On joining the Sisters of Charity, Joaquin had taken a vow of poverty, which meant that she earned only minimal living expenses all those years. The trustees were looking at an annual expense of some $60, 000 for another administrator—a considerable salary in the 1970s.

In her resignation letter of March 17, 1976, to Milo McGonagle, Chairman of the Board of Trustees, Sister Joaquin wrote:

> With this letter I wish to submit my resignation as President of St. Vincent Hospital, effective November 30, 1976...I am pleased that I can leave my successor a financially sound organization, and more importantly, a group of capable people in management positions....
>
> It has been a privilege to serve the community of Santa Fe and the northern area of New Mexico. I am proud to have had a part in legislation in this state that has helped health facilities throughout the state to serve the poor and needy and still remain solvent. These and many more are my memories of St. Vincent's and I am grateful for having been a part of its history.
>
> Sincerely, Sister Mary Joaquin, President

The indefatigable nun had accomplished what she had set out to do. She had turned the ownership of the hospital over to a nonprofit community corporation, the first of this kind in New Mexico. She relieved the Sisters of Charity of their $2 million debt, which would finally be paid when the Palace Avenue building was sold. She orchestrated the construction of a massive new nondenominational hospital for Santa Fe, located on a site that would allow for future expansion. And there would be room for the doctors to have their offices; the City had rezoned an adjacent 2.8-acre site for office use that would become the Medical-Dental Center. The hospital would soon find its new administrator in: Mikkel "Mike" Kelley. Kelley had held administrative positions at other New Mexico hospitals since 1961, and appeared well qualified to take the helm at St. Vincent's. Sister Mary Joaquin's services were no longer needed.

Sister Mary Joaquin's announcement that she would be leaving was greeted with mixed reactions by the hospital staff. According to *The New Mexican,* she had her detractors who felt that substantial wounds must be healed after years of battles. She stated that after the nurses formed the PPA, she had had no problem with the union. But the PPA disagreed: if there were no problems, some of the nurses argued, the PPA probably wouldn't exist.[12] In an April 11, 1976 interview with *The New Mexican,* a reporter asked the new president why she was considered controversial. Sister Joaquin replied:

> Why am I controversial? I think it's because I have had to fight every day of every year for money, for support, and for recognition to provide the basics to even keep this hospital running.... I've had to go to the legislature, to the Capitol, and into the community. I have never, never had the luxury of staying here in the hospital and serving merely as its chief officer.

The reporter commented that she has been described as "one of the toughest administrators of her type in the West." Sister responded: "And I guess I am. I'd rather have them say I'm tough, than have them describe me as a willy-nilly nun who can't solve problems. I've solved problems. You don't do that sitting behind a desk eight hours a day."[13]

While some on the hospital staff may have felt the sharp prick of that toughness, many on the outside realized its benefits to the hospital and to the community. *The New Mexican* titled its editorial: "Thank You, Sister." Commenting on the criticism of Sister Joaquin's determination and forcefulness, the editor noted, "There is no one, however, who would question her sincere desire to do what is best for the hospital or argue that during those sixteen years she has not devoted every bit of her time and energy in the community's behalf."[14]

From the community of Santa Fe, the announcement of her resignation unleashed a flurry of honorary awards. In July 1976, the Board of Realtors again awarded her "Citizen of the Year." Mayor Sam Pick proclaimed October 17 as the city's "Sister Mary Joaquin Day," awarding her at a dinner in her honor at the Hilton with a kiss and a city medallion, the latter reserved, according to *The New Mexican*, only for "Very Special People." Governor Jerry Apodaca cited her service to the citizens of the state of New Mexico, and presented her with a silver tray— which she promptly sent back to the Motherhouse in Cincinnati. The New Mexico Hospital Association gave her a special achievement award at a dinner honoring her service; the Capital Bank designated her their "community leader" and hung her portrait in the bank lobby; the Santa Fe Medical Society gave a dinner for her at the Inn of Loretto. The Board of Trustees sponsored an "appreciation dinner" with music by the Santa Fe High School Dance Band, and a humorous presentation by the emcee, which, according to T*he New Mexican*, brought the nun, alternately, smiles, laughs, blushes, and tears. One of the many gifts the trustees gave her at the dinner that especially delighted her, was a tape player with several cassettes of her favorite operas and classical music. The Hospital Auxiliary hosted a tea for her at the home of architect John Gaw Meem and his wife Nancy, at which the auxiliary gifted her with a round-trip train ticket to take a well-earned vacation to anywhere she wished to go in Mexico.

This last award was especially important. In the sixteen years that Sister Joaquin had been the CEO of St Vincent's, she had taken only two vacations. Both of these were with a group from the Santa Fe Opera Guild, of which she had been a member since coming to Santa Fe. Her friend, Marguerite Claffey, was her companion on these trips, and, given Sister Joaquin's vow of poverty, Marguerite had helped her with the cost. The first trip was to Rome, a city that Sister was eager to see, given her Italian heritage and her love of classical music. But there was a major problem. Sister Joaquin was afraid to fly, and there was no convenient way to get to Rome from New Mexico except by airplane. Her friends hit on the solution to the problem: they got her high on champagne before take-off, and kept her high the whole time the plane was in the air.

This method of panic-alleviation was followed for the second vacation as well. This time she went to the Adriatic, to the Yugoslavian cities, to the Greek Islands, and to Ephesus and Corinth to contemplate the cities of the Bible that Saint Paul had visited and where he had sown the seeds of Christianity in his letters to the people. Later she reminisced on the experience:

> At Ephesus there were the stone chairs for the judges who were questioning Paul, and at Corinth the market place at the well where Paul preached to the people.... At Delos a strange feeling came over me like 3000 years ago seemed like "today." I didn't feel I was in another age, I felt *connected* to all that was 3000 years ago.[15]

She delighted in swimming in the sea, and writes that she could see clearly fifteen feet to the bottom. And she was especially moved by the devotion of the Moslems at prayer in Istanbul's Blue Mosque. In 1972 she recounted these adventures in a letter to a friend in Cincinnati. In the same letter she reveals: "Almost lost my mind before I left.... [T]he havoc in our house this past two years is unbelievable." There had been trouble with some of the sisters spreading rumors and making nasty jabs at her. "We get the reputation of 'look how many are leaving St. V's,' but truth will win out in the long run and I am absolutely at peace, especially since the trip away from here." Some six sisters had left the hospital in the months immediately prior.[16]

In addition to having achieved her goal in regard to the new hospital, Sister Joaquin had another reason for resigning. She was sick. For years she had suffered from rheumatoid arthritis. No one knew this outside of a few close friends and her doctor, Bergere Kenney. Her pain was constant, but she managed to hide it. Her close friend, Marguerite Claffey, had moved up in the hospital hierarchy from gift shop volunteer to salaried director of public relations and administrative assistant. Marguerite appointed herself as cerberitic guard at the door to Sister Joaquin's office, often turning away people who wanted to meet with the administrator if she felt Joaquin was not feeling well. There were complaints that Claffey was a self-appointed barrier, causing considerable antagonism. Even Sister Ancilla, who was the assistant administrator of the hospital for two years in the early '70s, was often denied access to her boss. This was a curiously difficult situation for Ancilla. In the early '70s, the Cincinnati Order had appointed Sister Ancilla as superior of the Sisters of Charity in Santa Fe. Hence in her religious life, Sister Joaquin answered to Sister Ancilla as her superior, but in Sister Joaquin's role as boss of the hospital, Sister Ancilla answered to Sister Joaquin.[17]

Some eight months before Sister Joaquin resigned, her health began to further deteriorate. She developed connective tissue disease, a specific symptom of which is a condition called Raynaud's Phenomenon.[18] This condition affected the extremities of her body, a swelling and hardening of her toes and her fingers. She had started to wear gloves to keep her fingers warm. When she first came to Santa Fe, she had a piano in the basement of Marian Hall, but the rheumatoid arthritis had long since left her unable to play. And now the tips of her fingers were so painful, she could barely use a typewriter. Dr. Kenney felt that the disease was increasing because of the stress of her work. She had hoped that after she resigned, the problem would clear up. But it didn't. In April she wrote to a friend at the Motherhouse:

> "Two weeks ago, very suddenly, the right index finger got cold
> and has stayed cold. It is swollen all the time now, and I have
> two cracks in the skin at the tip, and it is as sore as an open
> nerve. The nail and finger are a light cyanotic color unless I am
> in the cold, and then it gets ghastly white. I saw Dr. Kenney....
> He doesn't indicate much else can be done."[19]

Dr. Kenney and other doctors she had seen all told her she must get out of her job and get to a warm climate.

Over the years, Sister Joaquin would sometimes escape from her office and spend a weekend in quiet and prayer at the remote Benedictine monastery, Christ in the Desert, some seventy-five miles north of Santa Fe. In 1964, Father Aelred Wall, a monk from New York, had founded the monastery in a spectacular high-desert canyon along the Chama River. He became a close friend and spiritual mentor to Sister Joaquin, but he left the monastery in 1973. He went to Mexico, where he built a hermitage for himself near the village of Los Rico some ten miles from San Miguel de Allende. He named his property Rancho de Nuestra Señora de la Soledad—referred to as just La Soledad. Aelred helped the impoverished villagers by starting a workshop to teach the boys and men to make furniture and various woodcrafts. Some of the things they made were sold in San Miguel and some were sent to be sold in shops in Santa Fe and Mexico City. The sales began to bring in money for their families. Aelred also developed a large flower garden and the villagers sold the flowers to the hotels in San Miguel. He helped the Los Rico villagers by providing doors and windows for their houses. His dream was someday to start a monastery on the property.

Shortly after Sister Joaquin submitted her resignation to the Board of Trustees in March of 1976, a letter arrived from Father Aelred inviting her to visit La Soledad and perhaps to consider joining him there. She did visit him, and they discussed the possibility of her building her own hermitage on his property. She knew her illness would improve in Mexico's warm air and she yearned for the chance to finally experience the contemplative life, which a move to Father Aelred's rancho promised. But at the time she wasn't in a position to consider such a move. She was worried that she didn't as yet have another job—as a Sister of Charity, she was expected to work for her living in some manner of social benefit. She couldn't just withdraw from her obligation to work to live a life of the spirit in Mexico. But her primary concern was to regain her health. Her health would dictate what turn the coming years would take.

6

~†~

*I*t must have been difficult for Sister Joaquin to witness the dismantling of Marian Hall. The convent had been her home and her place of worship for the last sixteen years, and it represented the presence of the Sisters of Charity in Santa Fe for well over a hundred years. The stained glass windows of the little chapel were removed and put into a small chapel in the new hospital. There were religious statues that were either to be given away to local churches or sold with the proceeds to go to the new hospital. Father Edward O'Byrne, the director of St. Vincent pastoral care, recalled a few years later that some of the pews and a small altar were moved to the new hospital chapel, and the main altar was given to St. Catherine Indian school. Although the new hospital would be nondenominational, pastoral care would continue to be provided by many religious groups. But the crosses that hung in every room of the Palace Avenue hospital would have to go. They could be placed in a patient's room in the new hospital only if requested.[1]

For Sister Joaquin, as well as for the many Sisters of Charity who had worked in the hospital over the years, there was sadness at ending their Order's association with St. Vincent's. After more than a century of service, it was inevitable both for financial and changing cultural reasons that the hospital should be turned over to the community. The sisters' hospital had played an important role in the city's history; the move to the new facility would bring that role to an end. Two of the four remaining sisters at the hospital, Sister Jane, the social worker. and Sister Mary Eudora from the business office decided not to leave after all, and to stay and work in the new hospital. The Marian Hall convent was now gone, but the two were able to find a home to "house-sit" on Old Santa Fe Trail. Sister Joaquin was pleased at their decision to stay in Santa Fe. She wrote to the provincial supervisor for the sisters in Colorado: "It is a wonderful thing having Sisters Mary Eudora and Jane stay on here....The Santa Fe community will be so happy, and it could mean the Sisters of Charity thread of service here need not be broken, but survive and grow." But the two women stayed for only two years.[2]

Sister Joaquin was determined to take a year of rest before she looked for another position. She was offered two good job opportunities in New Mexico: one with Presbyterian Medical Services as nursing supervisor in their Taos hospital and outlying clinics; the other as executive director of the state Health Systems Agency—these in addition to five offers from outside the state. But before she could consider committing herself to another job, she had to determine the long-term prognosis of her disease. In May 1976, she wrote to Sister Mary Assunta, who had previously been a nurse under Mary Joaquin at St. Vincent's, and now was the new president of the Cincinnati sisters:

> "I am really puzzled about God's will for me, when just as I was coming to some conclusions in my planning for my future, this strange condition in my hands gets suddenly worse, and it changes the outlook on everything.... [M]y deep desire (and it doesn't go away) of working somewhere and leading a more concentrated spiritual life, where the spiritual part does not take second place (or no place), is THE big thing in my life for the remaining years God has for me."

Sister Joaquin's concern to be free to pursue a spiritual life was as urgent as her need to find relief from her disease. She felt conflicted, in that her obligation to the Order as a Sister of Charity was to work "in the world." But the busyness and demands of such of work did not allow for a deep spiritual life, at least not for the kind of life she was craving. She continued in her letter to Mary Assunta:

"Right now I do not see anything I can do within the structure [of the Order] of the kind of life and work we do, that will answer this strong desire for more spirituality, less worldly, more concentration on what I can do for the world in the realm of sacrifice and prayer, as well as service. The present day life and work of our community is so noisy, worldly, and active that listening to the Spirit is nigh impossible."[3]

Sister Joaquin went to Cincinnati in June, to the Good Samaritan Hospital to get a further opinion on her health. The prognosis was again the same as that of the New Mexico doctors: the rheumatoid arthritis had led to mixed connective tissue disease with symptoms of Raynaud's Phenomenon and scleraderma. There was no known cure and no treatment available other than cortisone, which might give some relief. The recommendation was a move to the warm air of Phoenix or Tucson, San Diego or Mexico and remain free of stress for at least a year. After that, she should be tested annually to see if the disease was arrested.[4]

During summer and fall of 1976, Joaquin was unsure concerning her future. She was drawn to the idea of retreating to Mexico, to a life of quiet and prayer, yet she must earn her living in a manner that was within the expectations of her Order. Of one thing she was convinced: she had to find some place to rest and recover from the work demands of the last sixteen years, the stress of those years having at least contributed to, if perhaps not caused, her debilitating sickness.

The Hospital Foundation gave Sister Joaquin a car to use for a year and money for gas; the Cincinnati sisters approved her taking a sabbatical from any employment for a year. Tom Old, a charter member of the hospital's Board of Trustees, offered her a place to stay for a few weeks in Puerto Vallarta, where he owned two hotels. In late October 1976, Sister Joaquin and Marguerite Claffey went together to Puerto Vallarta.

Joaquin had taken a Spanish course in Santa Fe, but she had had little time to concentrate on learning the language. Marguerite, whose family reached back several generations in Hispanic New Mexico, did know the language. She helped Sister Joaquin settle into a small oceanfront apartment belonging to the Olds, across from Tom Old's hotel, the "Tropicana." Marguerite took Joaquin to the *supermercado* and explained to her how to buy groceries. She arranged for a friend of the Olds who taught in a nearby school to come and tutor Joaquin in Spanish. Then Marguerite returned to Santa Fe, leaving Sister to fend for herself.

Joaquin was delighted with her new surroundings. She was already making friends with the children playing in the street. They recognized her veil and immediately called her, *Hermana*. She acknowledged in a letter to Sr. Mary Assunta that although the world around her was incredibly noisy—traffic, children playing in the street, mariachis trumpeting from the hotel across the road—she was really enjoying the noisiness, at least for a while. It might not be conducive to contemplative prayer, but she knew she could find quiet later. For the moment she was absorbing a new world, a total change of environment from the stressful world of Santa Fe:

> I pray every day for the hospital, but it does seem far away, and I must admit I'm beginning to unwind. I still look at my watch often as if to check for 'next meeting,' 'next appt,' etc., etc., etc.... Maybe after a while I'll really learn to relax. I have complete privacy, and even though I miss the quiet, I do love to be with these simple people."[5]

Although she could not yet make any decisions about what she should do in the future, she had become convinced of one thing: she knew she wanted to be in a place that was full of the joy of children.

Sister Joaquin stayed in Puerto Vallarta until late in December. She worked on her Spanish and tried it out on the children and adults as she walked to church every day. She celebrated Thanksgiving dinner with Tom and Patsy Old, who had joined her for the holiday. She was impressed that Tom Old had caught a Spanish mackerel; fish and potatoes constituted their Thanksgiving feast. Everything seemed to be done in a different way in Mexico, and Joaquin found the differences refreshing.

The warm air of Puerto Vallarta was medicine to her body, except for the humid days. Her hands were the worst then—sore and swollen. She would still like to take the Presbyterian Medical Services job in Taos County, but she was unsure if she could stand the cold. The job paid a good salary, which she could send back to the Motherhouse, saving only a minimal amount for her own needs. She wrote to a friend, "I now know that if I don't take advantage of every day of this year to rest, pray, and exercise properly, there won't be a body to go to work. So I'm hard at it to at least stop the progress of the disease."[6]

There were yet more doctors to consult. Joaquin left Mexico to spend a month in Phoenix while she awaited the results from a number of tests; then to Cincinnati for more consultations and tests and to spend some time with her eighty-five-year-old Aunt Nelle in Wapakoneta—the first time in years she had been "home" for more than a couple of days at the most.

The doctors both in Phoenix and Cincinnati had recommended biofeedback to try to raise the heat in her body. At first Joaquin was skeptical, and dismissed the idea as too strange and remote. But when she returned to Santa Fe that Christmas, Dr. Kenney urged her to go to the Institute for Biofeedback in Tempe, Arizona. Dr. Elliott Wyloge, a friend who was formerly a radiologist at St. Vincent's, had become the director of the Institute. She agreed to return to Arizona and try it. Joaquin quickly became enthusiastic. With the help of the feedback monitoring machines, she learned to raise the temperature in her hands by ten to fifteen degrees. The sore ulcers that had started to form on the tips of two of her fingers from lack of blood disappeared. She began to realize that stress alone would turn her fingers white and swollen, and through the conscious mental control of her parasympathetic reactions in temperature, muscle and skin, she could send blood flowing to her fingers and toes. "You use your mind to its normal, but unused ability," she wrote to an acquaintance who was considering the treatment. In cases of rheumatoid arthritis, "stress constricts the muscles and the muscles clamp down on the blood vessels and impair circulation. I'm learning to reverse this process."[7]

She returned to Santa Fe with a sense of optimism that through the biofeedback process she could regain control of her health. She hadn't yet decided what she should do about a job, but she felt that God had led her to biofeedback, and He would show her the next steps to take. As she wrote to President Mary Assunta in February 1977, "God directed me… to biofeedback, which I knew nothing about. He will continue to lead me if I can stay open to His breathing in me. Somewhere 'out there' is my place to live, work and love for Him. That's all that matters."[8] In May, Sister Joaquin went to the Monastery of Christ in the Desert to celebrate the ordination of Prior Philip to the priesthood. She described the simple, austere celebration in a letter to Sister Mary Assunta:

> Archbishop Sanchez performed the ceremony, and Indians from San Juan Pueblo beat drums and chanted as the procession entered the church. Some three hundred guests and clergy gathered to witness the celebration, and the monks chanted the psalms in Gregorian chant.

She was profoundly moved by the celebration. She goes on in her letter to describe her condition during that visit, since May can still be cold in northern New Mexico:

> The first two weeks here were cold and my fingers and toes blanched and thumped and the tissue was beginning to break. I spent two days in my room as I could hardly walk. I was planning to leave when suddenly the weather cleared and got very warm and I'm a different person. When I'm warm and dry it's hard to think how bad this disease can get. I get to thinking I exaggerate it. But when the cold comes, it scares me how fast the reaction in my circulation takes place. My index fingers get almost dead in appearance and the pain is excruciating, like an open nerve in a tooth. Following an event like this my whole

body gets drained of all energy and it takes two to three days to get back to normal.... Sister Jane thought I should explain it more to you and Sister Mary Christopher so that you can understand why I'm trying so hard to find a climate I can live in and be able to work. I'm not just running around the country on a joy ride. Right now as I laboriously and slowly write this, my index finger is white as stone and painful. I've been doing the biofeedback treatments five to six times a day to try to get blood back in that finger.

Tomorrow, June first, I will go into deeper silence and solitude the remaining twelve days here. It will be a time of fasting as a penance as well as a supplication and one of deep communion with God in silence so I can hear His voice....I have great hope and trust in spite of the darkness at the present time. In about three and a half to four months the cold weather will again be upon us, and I'm hoping I have a warm dry place by then to live and work, if only on a trial basis.... The life of prayer, work, silence and solitude is still very strong in me. I don't know why it is there when each door I try seems shut. I've tried to put it away, to forget it, but it's always present, night and day. There's a voice that says, "come", but it seems God is playing games with me.[9]

While Sister Joaquin was in Phoenix learning the biofeedback techniques, she had stayed with friends in a religious community. The sisters' devotion to helping the aged and the poor, their loving generosity toward people in need, gave her a sense of peace and direction. "This whole atmosphere here," as she wrote to Sister Mary Assunta, "has brought peace and reason back to my torn mind and heart." In October her year of grace, supported by the Sisters of Charity, would be over; she had to come to a decision—and, as she had anticipated, God led her to that decision.

Although initially reluctant to give up professional opportunities, she now knew she could neither take the Taos job, which she had up until then seriously considered, or any other job in hospital work. She was determined to embrace the quiet, contemplative life that had been out of her grasp for all the stressful years in Santa Fe and for years before. She had yearned for peacefulness in her life, and she knew she must grab her chance now, rather than become involved in another full-time—-and for her probably debilitating—-position. Father Aelred had again urged her to join him at his rancho in Mexico, where workers from the adjacent village of Los Rico could build a hermitage for her. The villagers had no adequate health care, he wrote, and Joaquin could help them. She would be able to live the life she desired, and at the same time provide the desperately needed medical help to the people a few hours a week.

By this time it was clear to her that warm dry air either in the desert Southwest or in Mexico was essential to controlling her disease; there could be no question of working again in a cold climate. She was strongly drawn by the prospect of working with Father Aelred and sharing in his Benedictine life, and she knew that her nursing experience would allow her to help the people. She wasn't sure if living in very primitive conditions in Mexico might be too much for her physical endurance, but she was determined to try. She wrote Mary Assunta, "All I know is I must go back....God led me there, almost against my will, and He will not let me flounder."[10] First, however, she had a last bow to take in Santa Fe. She returned to oversee the final stages of the new hospital construction.

July 9, 1977 was the day of the move from the old hospital to the new. The move, itself, was a major community event. The City closed off Old Pecos Trail, and police with walkie-talkies were stationed at twenty-two intersections along the route from Palace Avenue to St. Michael's Drive, stopping traffic to allow ambulance convoys of patients with motorcycle escorts to pass. The exodus involved a fleet of a dozen ambulances borrowed from around the state and a small army of police, doctors, nurses, and other aides following in other vehicles. Huge trucks moved the hospital equipment to the new location. The ambulatory patients rode in cars and buses, accompanied by doctors. Two patients were moved from the intensive care unit and two from the coronary care unit. Ambulances were color-coded, indicating the condition of the patient being carried, whether life-support was needed, and where he or she should be delivered in the new hospital. General Electric supplied instruments to start the heart in case of cardiac arrest. The New Mexico National Guard had five helicopter crews on standby, and Los Alamos Medical Center was on alert to receive emergencies. Fully equipped emergency rooms in both the old and new hospitals were staffed during the move to maintain overlapping coverage for the community. Communications, directed by Dr. Robert Zone, were relayed through police command posts. The move had required months of planning and coordination with local and state agencies and other health facilities. The entire process was orchestrated by Trustee Chair, Mike McGonagle, and accomplished in twenty-four hours. There were no casualties.

The Palace Avenue hospital, constructed twenty-five years earlier, had cost $3.5 million. The final tally of costs for the new St. Vincent's came to $11,600,000 from municipal bonds, $3,700,000 in direct obligation notes, and $5,000,000 in grants and donations for a total of $20, 300,000. [11]

At the formal dedication ceremony of the new St. Vincent Hospital, Sister Joaquin was lauded by the doctors and staff, trustees and community leaders as the individual whose vision, hard work, financial savvy, and practical leadership had brought the new hospital into existence. The building, now with more than twice the floor space as the old one, was blessed by an ecumenical group of clergy, and the dancers from San Juan Pueblo performed a Buffalo Dance to "give thanks to the Gods for all they provide." At the close of the ceremony, everyone was invited inside to view the new facilities. Sister Joaquin went as far as the hospital door, but did not enter. In her quiet way she told the crowd: "My work here is finished." [12]

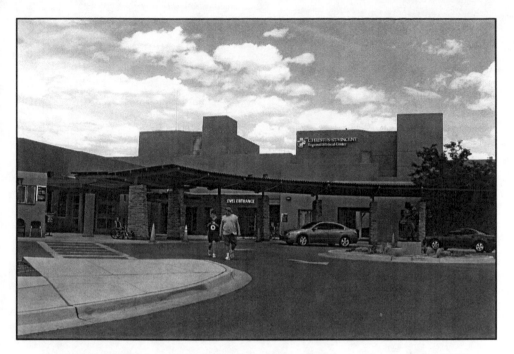

St. Vincent Hospital, opened 1977 on St Michael's Drive as it appears in 2009.
Photograph: Author's collection.

Part II

≈†≈

Rancho La Soledad.
Guanajuato, Mexico

> *The more one loses oneself in God,
> the more one becomes united with
> all creation.*
>
> —Sister Mary Joaquin

7

~†~

For Sister Joaquin to find a way to settle in Mexico, she first had to convince the governing board in Cincinnati that this was the right move for her, and that her proposal to provide medical assistance to the Mexican people merited the sisters' supporting her. Her plans for an eremitical life were not in concert with the usual activities the sisters were involved in: teaching, nursing, managing schools and hospitals, various kinds of social outreach. Generally, the nuns worked together in religious groups, as they had when serving at St. Vincent Hospital. These activities required active involvement in the local communities, activities for which the Order usually received income. Joaquin would, indeed, be offering medical help to the *campesinos* of the small adjacent village of some thirty-five families and to close surrounding settlements. There would be no income from this effort for the Order. The Sisters would have to support her in an endeavor that was somewhat marginal to their general program. She would have to do much fund-raising, especially among her Santa Fe friends. She would use her nursing skills to help the poor, but her greatest needs were to heal her own body and to lead a peaceful life of prayer.

Joaquin was blunt and forthright in her pitch for support to the regional superior, Sister Mary Christopher:

In the 34 years of my religious life I have never asked for any funds for a project or work. My work here at St. Vincent's was 17 years of trying to keep health care going for the northern people and the Santa Fe people, so many of whom are very poor. It was not an easy task. And the one big goal was to see that the Sisters of Charity were paid the debt Santa Fe owes them.... I have always worked without looking at the gain.... I ask you all to consider the above when you decide about helping with the funds.[1]

Late in October 1977, Sister Joaquin submitted her "Application for Overseas Ministry" along with a proposed budget to Sister Maryanna Coyle, the nun in charge of the Cincinnati sisters' ministry office. Her proposal stated:

As an outgrowth of a life of contemplation and prayer, three to four hours each day would be spent in visiting the homes of the rural poor in three villages, counseling and advising in nutrition and sanitation. The rest of each day would be spent in Eucharistic adoration, silence, and penance in keeping with the contemplative character of the life."[2]

Sister Joaquin's request for financial support was extremely modest, reflecting the sisters' maxim of "living simply that others may simply live." Her proposed budget for 1977-1978 for the initial start-up costs— construction of the hermitage, purchase of a car, gas, food, and travel expenses—was $10,500. She had already raised $5375 from her friends, and another $2500 was promised. So depending whether the promises were kept, she might need ask for only about $2500 from the Order. She also assured Sister Maryanna that her annual expenses after the initial costs would be far less.

Sister Maryanna was sympathetic to Joaquin's needs, both physical and spiritual. And since part of Joaquin's time would be spent in medical assistance to the poor, her proposal was certainly within the purview of the sisters' mission. Maryanna approved the ministry, but since it involved a request for financial support, she sent the application on to the Executive Council. Sister Joaquin was hoping for a quick response; Santa Fe would soon be getting cold, which meant she should leave for La Soledad no later than mid-November so that her hands would not swell and ulcerate again.

Joaquin had another reason to want to leave Santa Fe as soon as possible, as she wrote to her friend, Sister Annina: "The abortion issue is very 'hot' in town and I'd like to get away from the reporters, and the doctors, too. The trustees meet on Saturday at noon to approve or disapprove the vote of the medical staff, which voted FOR abortions…. This kind of 'hot' I don't need." The doctors' vote was thirty-two in favor, twenty-two against. The Board of Trustees overrode the vote: Abortions would not be performed at St. Vincent Hospital.[3]

The Sisters of Charity Executive Council approved the request for funds, and Sister Joaquin prepared to leave Santa Fe for a new life in Mexico.

~†~

Although Sister Joaquin looked forward to a solitary and peaceful existence in Mexico, she was hoping that perhaps one of the sisters might be similarly drawn to the contemplative life and would join her, at least for a few months. Not to share the same living quarters, but to talk and worship together in companionship, yet respecting the solitude of each. She repeated this wish over and over in her letters to Cincinnati. She wrote that she worried about being so marginal to her community of sisters and so isolated from them. Although she had chosen the contemplative life, a part of her missed the sense of community that participation in the activities of the Order meant to her. Joaquin, if a contemplative, was not a recluse. Many people commented on her outgoing warmth, her friendly smile. She had hoped that her close friend from St. Vincent's, Sister Jane might join her. Jane had wanted to, but she had other demands on her, and the other sisters either couldn't leave their jobs or were not interested in that kind of life.

La Soledad is some ten miles from the town of San Miguel de Allende and three miles from the pilgrimage site at the church at Atotonilco. Sister Joaquin found the land around the "ranchito"—as La Soledad was called by the locals—not unlike that of northern New Mexico, only greener, with valleys of alfalfa and gentle hills of cactus and mesquite. "It wouldn't be hard for me to have a Zen garden. The outcroppings of white rock look much like pictures of Greece. Mesquite trees look almost oriental, and there are a few poplars called *alamos*. But the earth is hard to dig and the mesquite for firewood is hard to cut."[4] A short distance away was the Laja River, an unpredictable element of the landscape that in some months could be a sluggish trickle, and in others a swift-moving course that was almost impossible to wade across. When the river was in full flow, even the horses and burros had trouble crossing. Given there was no bridge, wading was the only way for villagers to get from one side to the other, but from experience they were expert at balancing on the logs and knew where the stepping stones were located beneath the surface.

The village of Los Rico, across the river from La Soledad, was extremely poor. The population was a mixture of *mestizo* and Otomi—the latter an indigenous group from central Mexico that the Spanish colonists relocated from their home area near Mexico City. The Otomi were to be a buffer for the Spanish against the more belligerent indigenous groups, and later were enslaved to work on the farms and in the mines. There was much sickness in the village, and access to health care limited to nonexistent. The people lived in one-room adobes with dirt floors and no water or electricity. They were hungry much of the time, and if some of them even had shoes, the shoes were full of holes. Most families had from eight to fourteen children, and malnutrition was evident in the pinched faces, distended stomachs, and thin legs of the children. Alcoholism was also a major problem, causing the men to loose their jobs and hence their ability to provide for their families. These were the people that Mary Joaquin was determined to help.

Soon after her arrival, Sister Joaquin met a Mexican couple, Luis and Yerma Brito, who had been working as volunteer community organizers in the villages for several years. Luis was an ex-Jesuit seminarian, and both he and his wife were lawyers. The Britos would go to the peoples' houses and teach them planting methods and how to use the plants in the landscape around them, especially herbs for medicinal purposes. They organized farming cooperatives and instructed the people about sanitation and nutrition. The couple complained about Americans coming to the area, trying to be helpful by bringing their foreign medicines. The people would become dependent on the medicines, they said, and then the Americans would return to the States and the people were left without help. But the Britos responded to Sister Joaquin's friendliness and sincerity. They agreed to teach her to identify the medicinal herbs and to take her with them on their rounds of the villages so she could meet the people and determine their health needs.

The Britos invited Joaquin to Mass in the village of Galvanes, a small settlement some two and a half miles distant. The Bishop of Celaya, Victorino Alvarez, had been asked to celebrate Mass in the village that day. A visit by the bishop was an exciting event, and the villagers had strung crepe paper on the trees and bushes along the road to the church. Before the Mass, they set off fireworks, sang and beat drums, and rang the church bell to honor the bishop. After the ceremony, the Britos introduced Joaquin to Bishop Alvarez, and he warmly welcomed her to her new life in Mexico. He then officially introduced her to the people of the village. He explained that she would be helping them with their medical needs, and the villagers came and kissed her hands and the cross she wore around her neck.

Joaquin wrote to Mary Assunta at the end of December:

> I do keep a flexible but fairly regular schedule; I sing much
> of the Office—yes, by myself … spend time in reading and a
> special time for deep prayer. Often there are interruptions for
> decisions on the building, or by a mother and baby looking in
> my window, the mother holding up the penicillin to be given.
> But even the interruptions have a certain flow to them and they
> become part of my prayer.[5]

Thursdays and Sundays were visiting days at La Soledad, and tourists would sometimes leave a small donation to the "sick-poor" fund that Joaquin and Father Aelred set up. There were several Americans living in San Miguel, and many had wealthy guests from the States who would come and contribute. Father Aelred had had his friend, the architect George Nakashima, design and build a small chapel for La Soledad. The large altar table of a single piece of solid oak, Nakashima had brought from England, and his chapel design echoed that of a Greek village church. The celebrations of the Mass drew people from San Miguel as well as tourists and villagers to celebrate the holidays. Mary Joaquin was moved by the Mexican Christmas traditions, and described her first Christmas at La Soledad in a letter:

> *Farolitos* and *luminarias* were lining the path up to the chapel. There were a life-sized Joseph, Mary, and Jesus made of straw under the gazebo outside the chapel, and the people from Los Rico tethered several lambs, sheep, and burros right behind the crib. The people had built bonfires near the chapel, and hung tin lanterns with candles on the trees, As Father and the musicians proceeded up to the chapel singing the *Entrada* from the *Misa Americana,* people started coming out of the darkness into the candle light—beautiful Aztec faces with quiet but happy smiles, babies and old men and women. There were about a hundred villagers and some sixty Americans from San Miguel. So poorly clad serape-covered Indians stood next to fur jackets and suede suits. But everyone was comfortable. After the Mass (at the Gloria, they set off fireworks) Father served hot rum punch and Mexican cakes.[6]

The steady, contemplative life Joaquin was expecting had not yet settled in. During January, she planned to accompany the Britos Tuesday, Thursday, and Saturday evenings, take Spanish lessons with Josefina Vasquez in San Miguel on Mondays, Wednesdays, and Fridays, and spend the mornings doing chores and watching over the construction of her hermitage. She was very disciplined, ensuring time for herself in the mornings for reading and prayer, given that she rose every morning at 3 am to dress in time to recite the Divine Office with Father Aelred in his chapel. She expected to have improved sufficiently in Spanish by February that she could cut back on her lessons. She was staying in Aelred's guest house and was hoping that her own little hermitage—two 12 X 12 rooms with a bathroom in between and a kitchen in an L—would be ready soon so that she could move in and set up her clinic. She decided to call her hermitage Nuestra Señora de la Paz. The foundation was already poured, covering her Mother Elizabeth Seton medal she had buried beneath it, and half the needed 4000 adobe bricks were already drying in the sun. It was late for making adobes, October and November being the months when the sun was hottest in that part of Mexico, but Joaquin had been unable to get to Mexico earlier. A second tiny hermitage was being planned for visitors—Mary Joaquin was still hoping for a companion from among the sisters. As she watched the construction of her hermitage, which kept getting a later and later completion date, she recalled the psalmist's warning: *Unless the Lord build the house, they labor in vain that build it.* She had no doubt as to who was building her hermitage, but it seemed He was certainly taking His time. It was promised for the first of February, but then this was Mexico; Joaquin was still cleaning up after the workmen mid-April.

Mary Joaquin's first patient was an old Mexican woman with badly swollen legs and feet. Joaquin drove her to a doctor in town, got her medicated, paid her bill, and took her back to her home. Before long the social security hospital in San Miguel was sending her patients with their medicines for her to administer. She soon had no lack of patients—an abscessed tooth, a severe skin irritation, a heart congestion, babies with pneumonia. She was learning how abandoned the rural poor were, forgotten by their own government, living in adobe hovels with mud floors, no electricity, and their source of drinking water a polluted river.

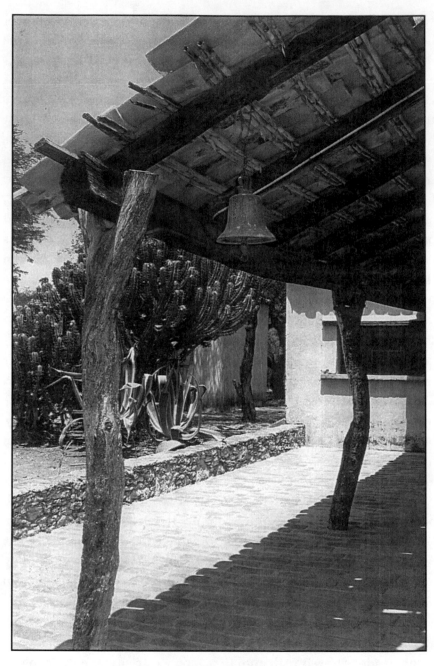
Mary Joaquin's hermitage, La Soledad.
Photograph: Author's collection.

Father Aelred preferred to call the life at La Soledad "monastic" rather than "contemplative." As in a monastery, there was much work to do besides prayer: *Ora et Labora*—prayer and work—is the Benedictine way. With rubber gloves to protect her sore hands, Mary Joaquin was able to work in the flower and vegetable gardens along with the *campesinos*. The gardens were part of Father Aelred's plan to help the villagers. The people sold the flowers and food in San Miguel, which gave them money to buy other kinds of food, clothes, and medicine—and, of course, alcohol. Joaquin also helped the men working in the woodworking studio, oiling the new furniture and art objects they made, getting them ready to sell. She felt her work to be part of her prayer—"working the earth and feeling the carved wood, [that are] part of His creation."[7]

Although Sister Joaquin had not yet been in La Soledad three months, the separation from her life in the United States caused her to see her home country in a different, perhaps clearer, light than when she had been so caught up in her work there. In February she wrote to Mary Assunta:

> "A land of plenty, but so materialistic it thinks it can do without God. May our country soon wake up before it destroys itself. So many warnings have been given the U.S.A.—our resources drying up, an atheistic youth, an unstable dollar … on and on. So much to plead before Our Father, and sacrifice for the needs of the unheard ones."[8]

Even though Mary Joaquin was feeling much better in La Soledad than she had for the last several months in the States, early in February, she got a warning as to her body's limitations in dealing with stress. Father Aelred had suffered a slight stroke, and Joaquin drove to San Miguel to get the doctor. Aelred's condition worsened over the next days and Joaquin sat up with him for three nights. After the third night of her vigil, she realized she couldn't endure any longer. Aelred would have to go to the hospital in Queretaro:

I could hardly move my hands [they were] so swollen and sore. I could barely hold a syringe without dropping it. Father was so weak I could not hold him up—no strength in my back.... I couldn't do another night, and Father would have to go to the hospital.... It's a sudden awakening to me—the progress this disease I have has made. I get the same reaction from stress as I do from cold.... The biofeedback exercises are a godsend. Without them I'm sure I would loose my right index finger as it always breaks down first.[9]

Every six months, Mary Joaquin needed to return to Santa Fe to see Dr. Kenney and renew her visa. She also needed to make contact again with the people who had donated funds to help start her clinic, and to try to find more donors. Her biggest expenses were gas for the car to take sick villagers to the doctors in San Miguel and Dolores Hidalgo, and to pay for their prescriptions if they had no money. Sometimes she had to pay for food and hospitalization as well, and twice in the first six months for two burials. In the six months after her little clinic was up and running, she treated 127 people, all from within a five-mile area. In a letter to Sister Maryanna explaining her need for more money from the sisters, she described a visit to one of her patients:

One young mother was too ill to come for her shot, so I went to her. Her husband led me down the three-quarter mile path and across the river on rocks and logs and up to her adobe. I stooped to enter a windowless 6 X 4 room with only a bed. I felt very humbled, but privileged to be here.[10]

Joaquin realized that she could not possibly meet the needs of all the villages in the vicinity of La Soledad. She tried to limit her service to just the villages of Los Rico and Galvanes. It meant turning people away, but she didn't have the money or the hours of the day to deal with all the problems that Mexico would bring to her door. This was extremely hard for her. She herself lived in great austerity, spending around a thousand dollars a year for her own needs, and much of that was the cost of her car. In addition to asking the sisters for funds, she wrote to donors asking for money to help the clinic. The clinic budget she submitted to Sister Maryanna for 1979 was for only $2000 with which she believed she could help six hundred people within a five-mile radius. She broke down the fund request as follows:

Medicine and supplies	$360.
Doctor services and prescriptions	$590
Hospitalization	$900
Food in special cases	$150
Total	$2000[11]

Sister Joaquin managed to get two small hermitages built and furnished with appliances and plumbing and local hand made rugs and furniture for under $8400—money she had received from her fundraising. Although she was glad that the sisters did not have to expend much money on her account, Joaquin actually felt that such a low figure for wages and materials was "tragic," given the dawn to dusk efforts of the workmen. It was an example of the labor situation in Mexico—wages that did little to alleviate poverty even when the people were working.

For the first time since Sister Mary Joaquin had joined the Sisters of Charity in 1943, she was able once again to have a dog. She had always loved dogs and had had a dog when she was a child, a fox terrier she reputedly shared licks with on her ice cream cones. But during her years working in hospitals and living in community with the sisters, there had been no room in her life for a dog. As soon as she arrived at La Soledad, Father Aelred presented her with a beautiful weimaraner that she named Nico. Aelred's dog, Chula, was of the same breed. Aelred told Joaquin: "Now you must sit down and talk to Nico.... [H]e is God's creation, and when you talk to Nico, you are praising God in His creation."[12] The villagers were amazed that Joaquin loved her dog so much that she bathed him—something they could scarcely believe.

Gradually over the spring and summer months, Father Aelred recovered from his stroke, and by October was on his way to St. Louis. He had grown up in St. Louis, and had friends there who were supporters of his workshop and gardens at La Soledad. He hoped to raise more funds from among his friends. He would be gone for six weeks, leaving Sister Joaquin alone with the two dogs for company. The two were good watchdogs and wonderful companions for her, but she was still disappointed that she did not have one of her sisters for a companion. She was resigned: "God knows best," she wrote in a letter to Mary Assunta, "and my hand is in His."[13] Father Aelred also left the Blessed Sacrament from the church for her to keep safe in her hermitage. She felt it a great honor to have such a holy object in her protective charge, to awaken in the night and see the flicking candle keeping vigil over her while she slept.

Shortly before Aelred's departure for St. Louis, Joaquin had a bad bout of flu with a high temperature. She had been treating several *campesinos* for flu the past weeks. She was careful about washing her hands well, but because of her own illness her resistance was low, and she, too, became sick. She recovered within a couple of days, but the flu had brought with it another jolt of awareness of her vulnerability. She wrote to Mary Assunta, that she felt "...my time in this environment, so one with the poor, is limited and that this disease is going to advance rather quickly. But it just makes me live more deeply in this life of prayer and apostolate before my time runs out. Thanks be to God and to you for allowing me to even be here."[14]

8

≈†≈

*I*n September 1978, Dr. Kenney wrote Sister Joaquin that he wanted her to return to Santa Fe for lab tests. It was important that she come at the latest by November because after that the weather would be too cold for her, and he didn't want her to put off testing for several months waiting on the weather. She had been in La Soledad for almost a year, and she had seen, as she put it in a letter, "the ground plowed, the corn planted, two harvests, and now the cutting and corn shucks."[1] She would leave as soon as Father Aelred returned from St. Louis, stay for a week, and hurry back to avoid the cold.

Joaquin was happy to see her friends in Santa Fe, and especially Marguerite Claffey at whose home she was always welcome to stay. She had sent ahead forty-five letters to possible donors, and was able to follow up on some of them in town. Her friends on the hospital Board of Trustees were elated because the state had finally purchased the Palace Avenue hospital building. Mary Joaquin was relieved. It was the final step of the transfer of $1.8 million still owed the Sisters of Charity. She had tried to negotiate the sale before she left for Mexico the year before, but the bureaucratic wheels couldn't be made to turn at her convenience. She was extremely concerned, however, that the decision, with her approval at the time, to hire Mike Kelley to replace her as administrator of the hospital, had not worked out well, and the trustees had had to let him go.

She left to return to La Soledad as soon as the lab reports were ready. They were not encouraging. She wrote to President Sister Mary Assunta to give her Dr. Kenney's report:

Dr. Kenny gave me a thorough checkup and exam, and said all is holding in what he calls a latent period.... My large toes have literally no flexibility anymore, and Kenny found the pulse over the instep very weak on the left and nearly gone on the right. I was really glad to get out of Santa Fe though when the temperature went down so fast. Days were 28 to 30 degrees and nights 16. When I get that cold I get dizzy, nauseated and extremely fatigued—almost like I'm doped. Here the days are 78 to 80 degrees, nights 50, but reaching 70 by 9 a.m. I feel so much better.

Her letter goes on to describe the situation in La Soledad at her return:

I wasn't back here two hours before two *campesinos* arrived with bad cases of the grip, and so the stream continued over the next week. I'm just short of 200 patient visits. One young man drove the prong of a rake in his upper arm and it left a nasty wound. He couldn't work so he had no food. He and his new wife asked me for help so I gave them 100 pesos to help until he could use his arm. When I went to bed that night I couldn't help thinking how many right across the river from me had not enough to eat. I'm glad I was driving [back to La Soledad] on Thanksgiving Day. I would find it hard to sit down to a big meal. Instead I sang all the songs I know praising and thanking God, and also prayed Americans would begin to realize that comfort and happiness and play are not the lot of millions on earth.[2]

By April 1979, she had to ask the sisters for more money. Since she didn't receive a salary for her work, she was dependent on a monthly maintenance check of $207 from the Order. The maintenance check was sufficient for her personal needs, but her sick-poor fund was based on donations, and fundraising had become more difficult. Without a subsidy, she told the sisters in her application, she would either have to cut down services, or use the money until the fund was depleted and stop altogether. The hospital in San Miguel wouldn't take the village patients unless Mary Joaquin paid for them. In her first year she had treated some 500 patients. The patients were equally men and women, and a third of all were children and babies. The patients exhibited maladies ranging from abscessed teeth to eye and ear infections, burns, diarrhea, malnutrition, extreme alcoholism, and just about every other scourge of humanity. A very ill patient in the States would be brought to the hospital in an ambulance; a sick patient from Los Rico would be brought to Sister Joaquin's clinic in a wheelbarrow. The governing board in Cincinnati honored Joaquin's request, and by August she had treated her 1000th patient.

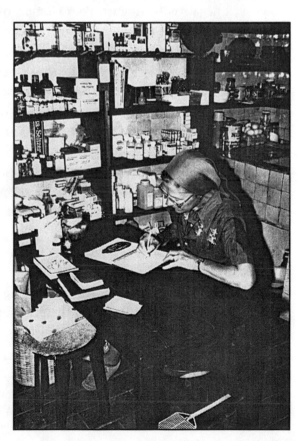

Sister Mary Joaquin in her clinic. Photograph: Sisters of Charity Archives.

In addition to her clinic work and her time of quiet and prayer, Sister Joaquin had many other things to concern her. One was Father Aelred, who had recovered from his stroke in January, but had also come down with hepatitis in June. She needed to keep a nurse's eye on him. She also had visitors from the States, although not the long-term companionship of a sister at La Soledad she would have liked. Her first visitor was Tony Taylor, brother of Lady Bird Johnson and owner of the Old Mexico Shop in Santa Fe. Tony's shop was a valuable outlet for the crafts made in La Soledad workshop. Marguerite Claffey came for a visit in May and drove Joaquin back to Santa Fe to renew her tourist card and to have a medical checkup. Then in June, her dear friend Sister Jane came, but only for a short stay. By mid-July, Joaquin was driving again to Santa Fe, this time worried she had caught Aelred's hepatitis, but the tests proved negative. In August, Polo Gomez, owner of the Artesanía shop in Santa Fe, came to order carvings and furniture from the workshop. Gomez was a good friend of Father Aelred, and had helped the monk build his monastery in New Mexico's Chama Canyon. By November Joaquin had again driven to Santa Fe to see Dr Kenney and do some fundraising. Sister Marie Vincentia visited for Christmas, and in January 1979, Prior Philip from Christ in the Desert monastery came to visit her and to celebrate the visit to Mexico of Pope John Paul II. The pontiff's messages were broadcast on the radio, and all during the week of his visit, Joaquin could hear snatches of John Paul's words coming out of the transistor radios that most of the *campesinos* carried as they walked by the hermitage to work or to town.

At the end of the year, Joaquin sent a report of her activities to the Sisters of Charity. She had managed to collect $2000 for the sick-poor fund during the three visits she made to Santa Fe during the year. This was only enough to take care of the people from Los Rico, and she had had to turn away people from other villages.

The people are very poor," she wrote, "and walk miles for their water—or worse, use the badly contaminated river water. There is no electricity in the village; the adults do not read or write, but their children now go to school by government order, to a school some two miles away, and some parents are learning from their children. Most of the *campesinos* do not have enough to eat most of the time. They suffer from a skin condition … which often makes painful cracks in their feet and hands a half inch deep. It's from unsanitary and dirty conditions."

She continues, writing that she had been able to help many men with the flu to stay in their jobs–if they were lucky enough to have one.

In Santa Fe, in addition to money, her physician friends donated medicines and basic medical supplies. She was also given clothes for the villagers. She brought back to La Soledad three carloads of clothing and could use much more:

Very early one cold morning (38 degrees) a woman came with her sick child. She was blue with cold, so I took a serape from the floor of the other hermitage and gave it to her. After I treated the *niño*, she went, all smiles, with the serape around her and the baby…. Yesterday I had three women and six *niños* from a nearby village. One baby was so ill—I did treat it, but tried to explain that I couldn't take care of people from all the surrounding villages…. As I watched them go over the hill, I felt so helpless, so lost as to what to do. They don't have access to even the barest of medical care, barely enough to eat, and no protection from the elements.

There is something to be said for leaving one's own land and people [to work] for the Lord. Living close to the poor in an underdeveloped country has an uncertainty about it that makes the whole venture a leap if faith. I really did not choose a foreign country, I was led to it in my search for a warm climate and solitude. There was an urge to go into the desert where there was no one but me and God, where reputation, talents, status and possessions mean nothing. There would be no supportive community, life would be stripped naked. I see the contemplative life here as natural.... But if the people lose their deep faith and mystic quality, we will have made them into our own image and likeness and I'm not sure the USA image and likeness deserve repetition.

Joaquin concludes the report with a description of the end of her day:

I go out on the portal under the stars and pray the Rosary for the Church, the Sisters of Charity, the Pope, the oppressed. I'm outdoors most of the day, close to the sky, the stars, the trees, the wind. That's when I think of God—me—life—Man—and as I get older I feel the shortness of this earthly pilgrimage, and I just hope and trust that what I'm doing is "making up for what is wanting in service to Christ Jesus" in some way.[3]

Clearly Sister Joaquin had much time to consider her role in trying in some small way to alleviate suffering, if it was only the sufferings of the people of one small village. But she was a member of a religious group whose mission it is to work to alleviate suffering on a much wider scale. And Joaquin was disappointed in the direction she saw the sisters, as a community, moving: away from selfless giving, away from sympathetic caring and toward self-conscious intellectualizing and analysis, forming too many statements and resolutions. In December 1979, she wrote to Sister Helen Flaherty, the newly elected president of the Sisters of Charity:

After reading the *Catholic Telegraph Supplement* [a publication of the archdiocese of Cincinnati] I come away with grave concerns—concerns about what our Community is doing and where it is going.... While the ministries of great need are before us, we fan the flames over self-interest issues like women's rights, ordination of women, secularism, and on and on. While one woman leads her community in other corners of the world, [those she leads] are humbly, quietly, simply giving of themselves to the basest of the basest of humans. Her work has mysteriously reached out to millions, and recently to the highest professionals in our land and given the Nobel Peace Prize. Mother Teresa is like Saint Thérèse [of Lisieux] who, without leaving her convent, reached out to lives of thousands to raise them up. God has put into woman more compassion, more "feel" for finding the destitute and suffering, more love and warmth –this is what a woman is. We women religious will make a difference in our ministries by love and concern and action for those suffering. Why we have to be so caught up with "partnership," "equality," etc. in the Church puzzles me. Mother Teresa has demanded respect of the highest Church officials because she's not looking for it…. She has no time to spend in discussions about "how I can be more in the Church hierarchy"…. The world shouts for love and service from us, and in its spiritual hunger, reaches out to those who live the love of God in all they do, humbly and poorly."[4]

Sister Joaquin had not changed her attitude toward the contemporary concerns of women in all walks as to their role within a male-dominated society, yet she worried that in writing her thoughts to her Community, that she would be "scoffed at and ridiculous." In her position as hospital administrator, she was considered by the male business establishment to be a brilliant businesswoman. And yet to the reporter who asked her if her position was a symbolic victory for women's "lib", she had responded: "what do they want to be liberated from, their womanhood?" Clearly, she saw the role of women, especially the role of women religious, as independent of male striving for position. The woman will gain the respect of society by being herself, with all the warmth and care and loving that Sister Joaquin attributed to her, and which she herself tried to carry out in her ministry to the poor and sick at La Soledad.

Joaquin was not only concerned about the attitude of the women of the Church. Later, in a letter to Prior Philip of Christ in the Desert, she wrote:

> As I read the *National Catholic Review* and the *Cincinnati Telegraph*, it seems the Church is really suffering from defections and dissatisfaction with John Paul. So much protesting and harsh words, and the issue of Liberation Theology, the Nicaraguan thing, and on and on. Do you think that all this is to let the rigidity, pomp, and majesty of the hierarchy blow up, disintegrate or something so that "the Church" can become more simple, poor, and holy?[5]

Perhaps her work at La Soledad was the answer to her own question.

9

~†~

For the next five years, Sister Joaquin's life at La Soledad continued much as it had since she started the clinic in 1978. Mornings were reserved for prayer and contemplative reading, afternoons were spent treating the villagers at her clinic. The clinic consisted of several cupboards full of bandages and antibiotics, as well as vaccines and other serums she kept in a gas refrigerator—a contraption that stank of burnt carbon when it iced up, and which frequently threatened to quit on her with the consequent loss of expensive medicines. During the clinic hours—afternoons from two to five—her patients would line up on the low wall along the portal to wait their turn. Occasionally she would cross the river on stones and logs to the village to check on her patients and their living conditions, but this was difficult for her. Generally she expected her patients to come to the clinic. Worried about losing their jobs, most patients would wait to come until their symptoms were severe. "Sanitation is so bad," Joaquin told a reporter, "that one doesn't know where to begin. They know about boiling water, but they don't always do it. And they'll skip the last two shots if a sick baby seems better; so of course, the trouble occurs again."[1] The ranchito at La Soledad had a well that served the hermitages, yet Mary Joaquin always boiled the water she used for drinking and washing vegetables. She was very disturbed at the amount of alcoholism among many of the village men, causing them to lose what jobs they were able to get, with the consequent impact on their families. Father Aelred's workshops and gardens helped some of them get money for their families, yet once they were paid, too many of them spent their earnings on drink.

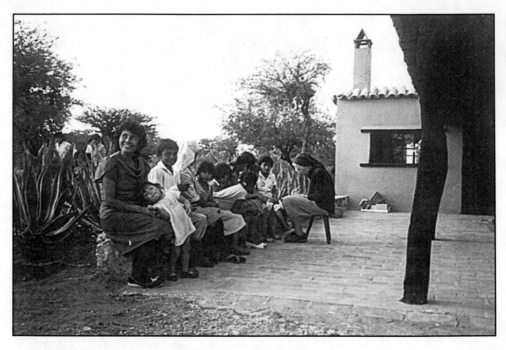

Patients await their turn, seated on the stone wall.
Photograph: Deborah Douglas collection.

Shortly after Father Aelred had initially settled at La Soledad, Luis Brito, the Jesuit-educated rural economic, health, and nutrition advisor who worked in the surrounding villages, had been told of the priest's establishment. He decided he must meet this American *padre* who was trying to help the people. Brito described his first meeting with Aelred, and the initial effect on him of that meeting.

The road stops 300 meters from a small house composed of three rooms of simple and lovely construction. We decided to shout to establish communication with the monk: Padre Wall! Padre Wall! Padre Wall! A tall man with white hair and a blue habit accompanied by a weimaraner dog came toward us. We truthfully had an experience of peace. For the first time in my life I felt the peace—this animated state where there is no time, no hurry. The sensation was as if tranquility enveloped me. It was a great gift. It was clear we were in the presence of a man of God. He was interested in our social labor, and he told us that for him the awakening of the secular was the way God is present in this world.

Brito and the Benedictine monk became good friends. Luis helped Father Aelred by taking some of the artisans to Mexico City to sell their goods. He goes on in his account to lament the problems of the *campesinos'* drinking:

I accompanied Padre and two of the artisans to Mexico City to make sales agreements with the idea the *campesinos* would understand the agreements. The pieces that they produced were of such a quality that the artisans were able to make several sales agreements, and they were delivered money in advance. Padre returned confident the men understood the agreements, but they got drunk and caused argument and sadness. To our way of thinking this disillusionment accelerated the damage or loss of Padre's health, so that on an occasion when we visited him we found him in bed in a critical state. He told us that in case of his death, he hoped we would continue his work.[2]

Sister Joaquin was constantly worried about the villagers' drinking. She would take one of them into San Miguel each Sunday to an Alcoholics Anonymous meeting. Father Aelred seemed to have more influence over them than she did. In a letter to Prior Philip at Christ in the Desert she wrote that she was nervous that Aelred was away in New York for two weeks, and she hoped that the villagers would stay sober. "Two weeks ago [one of the men] in the village, pressured [his neighbor] to take a beer, and that did it! He was very ill for five days. It's so sad when *all* his neighbors and friends are alcoholics. The pressure must be awful!"[3] Joaquin had good reason to be nervous about being alone at La Soledad. More than once there was a knock at her door in the middle of the night by someone inebriated. She would not open her door to such a late intrusion unless it was a woman who was seeking her help in an emergency.

One November day in 1984, shortly after Father Aelred's return from New York, Sister Joaquin was surprised that Aelred's dog, Chula, did not come to greet her as she did every morning. She went to check on the monk, and found him on the floor, toothbrush in one hand, toothpaste in the other. His mouth was twisted to one side, and she knew immediately he had suffered a fatal stroke. She went to town to bring a doctor to write a death certificate, and when she returned she found fifty *campesinos* around him, praying the rosary. All night and all day for two and a half days, the villagers came and went, bringing flowers and prayers. Brother Philip and Brother Francisco from Christ in the Desert, the monastery that Aelred had founded in the Chama Canyon of New Mexico twenty years earlier, came to celebrate the funeral Mass. Father Aelred's family arrived shortly, and at the funeral there were over a hundred from the villages and well over a hundred other Mexican and American friends. "The mariachi group who always sing and play the *Pan American Mass* at Father's Christmas Midnight Mass played for the funeral," Sister Joaquin wrote to the Sisters. "It was joyful and very beautiful—musicians, cross bearer, priests, family and friends processing up the hill to the chapel."[4] Aelred was laid in a simple wooden casket, his body wrapped in a woven Mexican blanket that Sister Joaquin had chosen. He was buried a short distance from his hermitage among some mesquite trees, his grave marked by a wooden cross his workers made for him: *20 V 1917 - Padre Elredo Wall - 13 XI 1984 Monje de Monasterio de Cristo en el Desierto.* They protested that the wooden cross was not worthy of him, but it was the best they could do.

Shortly before his death, Father Aelred had willed La Soledad to the Benedictine brothers at Christ in the Desert. Sister Joaquin, too, had received permission from the Cincinnati Sisters to transfer ownership of her hermitage to the Chama monastery. However under Mexican law at the time, neither religious communities nor foreign individuals were able to own real property; hence there were problems with the will at Aelred's death. Since he was not the legal owner, he could not bequeath the property to the New Mexico monastery, which also could not be a legal owner. The title to La Soledad was held for Father Aelred by a Mexican friend, Teresa Lamas, in San Miguel. To comply with the law, an *asociación civil*, a nonprofit corporation for the manufacture of handmade furniture and art crafts was formed.[5] The *asociación civil* was composed only of lay people, and remained the legal owner of the property for several years until the law was changed to permit the creation of an *asociación religiosa,* and the title could be transfered to the monastery. The brothers asked Mary Joaquin to stay on at La Soledad and continue her work with the clinic.

Father Aelred had started construction on a school for the Los Rico villagers, with Edward Meyers of Albuquerque the architect and director of the project, but the school was not completed before his death. By the next July, however, the school was finished, and Prior Philip along with many benefactors came to La Soledad to participate in the blessing of the new school. Thirty children were admitted to the first and second grades, including some ten to fourteen-year-olds, who had never started school. The school also offered literacy classes for teenagers and adults. The teacher was provided by the Education Department of the State of Guanajuato. The New Mexico monastery sent two monks, Brother Francisco and Brother Christopher, to live the monastic life at La Soledad and prepare to found a complete monastery. They were to take care of the property, assist with the workshop, and minister to the villagers. They also helped Joaquin with the food program she had started with the help of a church group from St. Maurice Parish in Florida, a parish that sponsored several hunger programs for the poor. The program provided milk, rice, cheese, and iron-enriched rice flour to the villagers.

Sister Joaquin grieved at the number of little white coffins that were carried in procession to their burial. As a devout member of the Catholic Church, she had always loyally followed the strictures of Rome. But her experience with the sufferings of the villagers had changed her in one respect. She no longer believed that the Church's edicts regarding birth control were valid. Some of the village women of Los Rico had as many as fourteen babies. These were babies the family could scarcely afford to feed, and many of them soon occupied the little coffins—dead of infantile diarrhea or the many parasitic diseases brought on by the wretched conditions in which they had struggled for life. Joaquin was determined to help the women. She secured Depo-Provera, a birth control agent that had recently come on the market, an injection of which would hinder conception for 90 days. With the women's permission, she began inoculating them on a regular basis. "I don't care what the Pope says," Joaquin told some friends in Santa Fe. "These women needed help." What could be God's will in countenancing death after death of these babies?[6]

Mexico could be a very dangerous place, especially in the rural areas. A story that Sister Joaquin related to friends in Santa Fe brought this home. One day when Joaquin and Brother Francisco were driving in a remote area, they were stopped by armed banditos. "I knew this was the end," she said. "One doesn't survive these attacks." Brother Francisco pulled out a cross from under his shirt and waved it at the attackers: "*Soy cura!*" he shouted at them (I am a priest!). The banditos fled, confirming that fear of the Lord is the beginning of wisdom.[7]

With the monks' help, Sister Joaquin was relieved of some of the work involved at the ranchito, and this allowed her the time to give consideration to other needs of the people. By the 1980s, Joaquin was treating some 2000 patients a year, many of those being repeat visits. The task she felt the most important was to develop a source of clean drinking water. Besides washing in the polluted river, the villagers were drawing water from a two-foot hole near the riverbank that was filled by seepage from the river. The water was carrying sewage from upstream villages; hence the water hole was just as polluted as the river itself. The alternative was for the women to walk two miles for clean water. Infant deaths, especially from amoebic dysentery, were all too common. Sister Joaquin determined that a well must be dug to provide safe water for the village.

Early in 1985, on one of her many trips back to Santa Fe, she spread word in the newspaper that she was looking for donations to provide for a well for the village of Los Rico. Members of the First Presbyterian Church of Santa Fe read about her fund drive, and the church's environmental committee decided to take on the project. David Douglas, an environmental lawyer and chair of the committee, went to La Soledad to meet Sister Joaquin and investigate the situation. He returned to Santa Fe convinced of the necessity of the project. It would be of a small enough scale that the church members, along with donations from the community, could take on the funding. They were excited that they could really make a difference in the lives of the people. Joaquin estimated that the cost of the well would be about $10 - $11,000 dollars, but at the time the peso was frequently being devalued, hence it was not possible to make a firm estimate. The community-wide campaign, spearheaded by Douglas, raised enough money, but it took some time.

Building a well in Mexico was not a simple matter. There were many questions: where should it be drilled and how deep the expected water level; what kind of rock might be encountered; what kind of pump to use—windmill? gasoline generator? solar? If the energy were wind, how many hours of the day would the wind blow and at what speed? If solar, how many hours of sunshine could be expected? What kind of pipe—plastic or iron? What diameter? How many gallons per hour would it have to pump? How far would be the vertical lift—the distance the water would have to travel up the well to the surface and then up to a holding tank? What would be the minimum amount of water each household would need? Whatever pump was determined the most cost effective, it should also require only minimum maintenance so that the villagers themselves would be able to take care of it in the future. How many faucets should there be in the village, and where should they be located? Where to buy the parts once it was decided the best route to go? Parts sent from the States could be held up a long time in customs, and in the past there had been stories of exorbitant duties imposed; parts bought in Mexico might or might not be adequate.

And then there was the Mexican bureaucracy: the necessary drilling permit, possible *mordidas*, timing—getting all of the components together on site at the same time, along with the workers and engineer. Agreed-upon appointments were notorious for being missed. Some in the bureaucracy could be helpful; others couldn't care less—as some expressed about a well permit for a bunch of *campesinos*. Laborers must be hired. A committee of Los Rico residents must be organized to be responsible for the well during the installation and once it was in operation, and there needed to be a local villager as *mayordomo* in charge of the well.

There were phone calls back and forth to the States; money had to be raised and sent through bank drafts. Consultants had to be consulted on all of the above matters, both in the States and in Mexico. Joaquin had frequent consultations with David Douglas, by mail—which could take two to three weeks to arrive, if it wasn't lost or confiscated—and by many trips to San Miguel to use the telephone. Douglas was in constant negotiations with purveyors of well drilling equipment, all of whom had different ideas on the best way to proceed. In addition to funds contributed from members of the First Presbyterian Church and funds raised in the community, Sunwest bank pitched in the price of a compressed air windmill, and took charge of the donated money, sending drafts in pesos to San Miguel. Visitors to La Soledad left contributions. Lawrence Rockefeller, who had been a friend of Father Aelred, came to visit his friend's grave, and later sent a sizeable donation.

The Los Rico villagers elected four members to the water committee to represent them, and chose Florentino Ramirez as their *mayordomo,* the man who would continue to maintain the project after it was operational. The role of the committee was to be the voice of the villagers in dealing with the bureaucracy, it was important that the well not be seen as an American-sponsored charity project. Once the well was in place, it would also be up to the committee to collect the few pesos from the water users every month to pay for ongoing maintenance.

Joaquin also made trips back to Santa Fe to discuss the situation with Douglas and others involved in the project and to continue to raise funds. At one point, a chain saw was needed. Deborah Douglas, David's wife, drove Sister Joaquin back to Mexico with the chain saw hidden in the back of the car under a blanket. They made it across the border without the saw being discovered, hence not having to pay a duty on it—or worse, having it confiscated. A little further on, Joaquin asked Deborah to stop. She got out and said the *Te Deum* by the side of the road in thanks to the Almighty for letting them get the chain saw safely across.

In an article, titled "Border Crossings," written some years later, Deborah Douglas described an experience at the Laredo border crossing with Sister Joaquin:

> The US/Mexican border at Laredo may not be as mythically dreadful as the gates to the Underworld described in the *Aeneid*, but the scowling uniformed guards, with their dark glasses and their guns, reminded me of Cerberus (although I refrained from telling them so.) Madre [the name the villagers gave to Sister Joaquin] was completely unruffled during the ordeal of customs, serene and expressionless as they searched the car and barked questions in Spanish about her identity and authorizations. "And who is this one?" I knew enough Spanish to understand the immigration officer's demand, as he reached for my passport.
>
> "*Ella es mi compañera*," Madre calmly replied. She is my companion. I felt honored by this designation, which seemed to include me in her vocation—which probably nudged me a bit closer to some interior borders of my own.[8]

Sister Joaquin's knowledge of Spanish was never very extensive, consisting primarily of words relating to diseases and medicines and those necessary for dealing with the barked questionings of border guards. Some of the negotiations for the well were taken on by Christ in the Desert's Brother Francisco, who was fluent in Spanish, and had come to La Soledad to help with the property. The delays were myriad. In a letter to David Douglas on October 24, 1985, Joaquin wrote:

When I returned October 5th [from Santa Fe], I expected to see the drilling machinery at Los Rico. But no, it was about a mile downriver from Los Rico, drilling a second well for a neighbor. I'm sure you are familiar with the Mexican trait of leaning toward people of influence. That's what's occurred. However, in this interval, there have been two meetings of the people (men and women) from Los Rico. They elected four men to be the committee for the well. These four will now go to Celaya (for the third time) to get the permit papers. The last 2 times they went they were told another paper was needed. They've been to the *Municipál* four times and each time were told what to do—only to have the engineer in Celaya say *another* paper was needed.... Brother Francisco will go with them this time to see if he can help.... The well-to-do Mexicans don't care much about their needy brothers and sisters in this country, and the *campesino* is so used to it, he just takes it as a matter of course as he has no power.[9]

With the fluctuation in the peso exchange and the rising prices of Mexican goods, Sister Joaquin was having difficulty keeping accounts of the anticipated costs. She wrote to David Douglas in early November, 1985 that in July, $1000 US exchanged at 300,000 pesos, and a sack of cement was 800 pesos. Three months later, $1000 exchanged at 440,000 and the cement was 1570 pesos. And of course, the costs were increased by the seemingly endless waits on the bureaucracy, the well driller, the missed appointments, and the officials adding the need for signatures on paper after paper. Not to mention the days of lost work by the emissaries' fruitless trips. The engineer from Celaya at the *Registro Hidrolicos* didn't want to bother to come out to Los Rico, so he asked Florentino for 4000 pesos as *mordida*, so that no questions would be asked.... "Can you believe it?" Joaquin wrote Douglas. "And he's on a government salary—ugh!!"[10]

The situation wasn't much better by the next February 1986. On the 26th, Sister Joaquin wrote to Douglas that the windmill, which was sent down from the States in December, was still at the Mexico City airport. She had placed two 30-day restraining orders on the mill so that it wouldn't be confiscated. New papers had to be drawn up because the man who signed the papers for the windmill in early January was removed from office, hence Joaquin had to start all over again. The well permit was in some office in Mexico City and was supposed to be sent to Celaya, but after several calls to Celaya, the permit still hadn't arrived. The well driller did a sloppy job, not digging it as deep as Joaquin had specified. When she complained to him, insisting he dig it correctly, the response was, "Madre, why do you care so much about these people? They're just peasants."

Bill Halloran, an engineer from El Paso and a friend of the New Mexico monks, took charge of installing the pump, supervising construction of the storage tank, and providing the distribution system for the village. Halloran volunteered his time, and Sister Joaquin paid for the materials. The villagers had agreed to dig the trenches for the pipes on their days off from work at no charge, but the pipes weren't available, and Joaquin was still searching around for another supplier. The pump was to be sent from Monterey in ten days, but more than two weeks later there was still no pump. By this time, a year had passed since the project first started. "No wonder the poor get nothing done," Joaquin wrote. "Everyone just ignores them. They wait and wait in those government offices as the more well-to-do pass in and out in front of them."[11] In an April 29th letter, Joaquin wrote Douglas that the well was dug, the trenches and pipes were in to the village faucets, and they were ready to test the water. But the windmill was not yet up, and they still had not received the permit. In a May 7 postscript update, Joaquin reported that Florentino Ramirez, the *majordomo*, was *again* on his way to Celaya to try to get the permit.

By June 1986 there was clean water in Los Rico. Watching the water come up for the first time, the villagers cheered. There were a few details left to do, such as yet secure the elusive well permit, but the windmill was finally set up, and the water flowed into four faucets spaced around the village. There were plans to perhaps later build a bathhouse, and maybe someday to have faucets in each house; but for now it was celebration time. There wasn't any beer or rum, because of the alcoholism in the village, just *refrescos*—Sister Joaquin was determined that it would be a happy celebration. And it was, with blessings for the well by clergy and delighted children playing in the water.

When all the expenses were totaled, the project had cost $9,500, with a few dollars left over from the donations. These went to Luis Brito, to start a well in another village. Mary Joaquin and a friend took a long vacation to Florida.

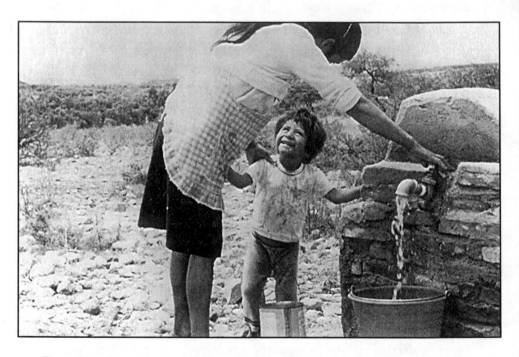

The well water arrives in Los Rico. Photograph: Deborah Douglas collection.

10

~†~

E ven with the clean water available, there was still much educational work to do. The people, especially the children, were still suffering from dehydration, and dehydration from diarrhea was the chief killer of children across Mexico. Ironically, dehydration is often caused by the water itself, just as malnutrition may not necessarily mean lack of food, (although that was still a problem in Los Rico) but the inability to assimilate the food's nutrients—again because of contaminated water. The cases of dysentery and other water-borne parasitic illnesses gradually declined at Los Rico, but Sister Joaquin had to constantly remind the villagers to be careful. Even if the people drank only the clean well water and bathed and washed their food in clean water, sometimes the pails used to carry the water might be contaminated, and in the hot summer, the children would play in the river—easy prey for parasites. Again and again the infections would recur. Mary Joaquin realized that it might take a generation for the people to change their ways from how they had always lived. But she was happy that at least there were fewer little coffins being carried to the village church than before the advent of the well.

After all the trouble involved in securing the windmill from the Mexican customs, it soon proved inadequate, and had to be replaced by a gasoline pump.[1] But the success of the well project at Los Rico spun off several other projects along the Laja River. Luis Brito, again with the help of members of the First Presbyterian Church of Santa Fe as well as other church organizations, raised funds for wells in four other villages. The Los Rico well also served as an inspiration for David Douglas to establish a nonprofit organization, which he calls "Waterlines." In the years that followed, Douglas's Waterlines would sponsor many water projects in third world countries.[2]

Now that the well project was completed, Sister Mary Joaquin had yet another project in mind for the village of Los Rico: a bridge. In warm weather, the Laja River was low, and easily traversed on logs and stepping from stone to stone. But during the rainy season, the river might be almost waist deep, and the little children had to be carried across in their parents' arms. Mary Joaquin discussed the possibility of building a footbridge across the river with Ed Crocker, a Santa Fe engineer who had been a key consultant on the well project. Crocker agreed to supervise the project, but insisted that the work crew be made up of men from the village. Joaquin and Brother Francisco found the cable and the pipes for the pilings and organized the village workers. Sister Jane raised funds from among the sisters at the Motherhouse. Crocker knocked on doors in Santa Fe asking for funds for the project. He was pleased with the response: "I was only turned down twice," he reported.[3] With a donated 1978 Nissan station wagon and two Santa Fe students, Crocker arrived in Los Rico in January, 1987. Twenty-eight villagers had agreed to help build the bridge, digging the holes with picks and shovels for the pilings to anchor the cables for the three-foot wide, 150-foot span. The floor of the bridge was steel mesh covered by wooden planks and the sides were chain link. While the cement on the pilings hardened, the crew went upstream to dig a diversion channel in case the river should overflow its banks, and planted river cane along the channel to hold the sides from erosion. Over the years the cane has spread, still protecting the riverbank. Brother Francisco was the "bridge" between Crocker, who donated his time, and the workers, who donated theirs; Sister Joaquin was the "enforcer." Francisco recalled, "If someone would not work, they would get no help from Sister."[4]

With the final tightening of the cables, the project was complete. Unlike the year and a half it had taken to finish the well project, the new bridge had taken only two weeks to construct. The village celebrated the new bridge with a fiesta. The children presented a dance they had worked on, and the bridge was decorated with balloons and colored streamers. There was plenty of chile, beans, and tamales for everyone.

Before long, however, Mary Joaquin noticed that the wooden planks on the floor of the bridge were gradually, one by one, disappearing. She realized that they were being taken for firewood. Over the years, the villagers had cut down many of the trees in the area, leaving the landscape eroded in areas. There wasn't anything she could do about the ecological problems the people had created for themselves in their need for fuel, but she salvaged the bridge by replacing the floor with layers of tight iron mesh.[5]

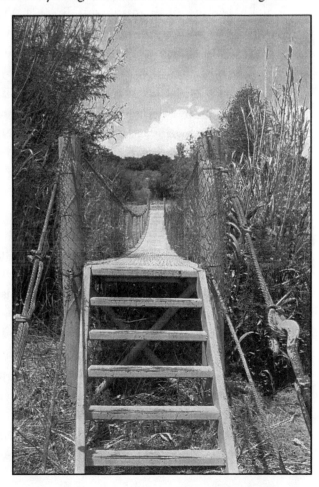

The villager's bridge over the Laja River. Photograph: Author's collection.

While the well project was underway, Sister Jane finally came to live at La Soledad as Joaquin had hoped for so long. Jane continued again her social work with the people of Los Rico as she had helped Joaquin at the hospital in Santa Fe years earlier. Before the bridge was built, Jane was afraid to cross the river on the logs, so she would stand at the river's edge and call to the children to come and take her hand to help her across. Since Jane was fluent in Spanish, she helped Brother Francisco teach the catechism to the villagers, and she also helped out at the school. Her friendliness, as well as her ability to communicate in Spanish, created a good rapport with the people, and allowed many of them to open up to her and discuss their problems. Jane also gave Joaquin lessons in Spanish, and Brother Francisco taught Joaquin to chant the psalms for the Divine Office in Spanish along with the villagers, who occasionally came to the service.

The dog, Nico, that Father Aelred had given Joaquin suffered from arthritis, just as did his owner. Nico didn't survive long, and in 1986 Joaquin was given a twelve-week-old puppy, Fortunata, or Nata for short. Joaquin was both delighted and overwhelmed. Nata was a smart little pup, but she was a pup—chewing everything, running off and getting lost, as pups tend to do. So to add to her duties managing the clinic and making hospital runs to San Miguel, hassling the problems dealing with the well and the bridge, worrying about the Mexican bureaucrats with their delays and their *mordidas*, worrying that the workers might show up drunk or not show up at all, Joaquin's time was also taken up with dog training. In this, Brother Francisco tried to help, but with his responsibilities in the monastery and his pastoral work with Sister Jane, he didn't have much time for dog training. Brother Christopher couldn't be bothered— definitely *not* a dog person. Aelred's dog, Chula, was quite offended at first, snapping and barking at the intruder. Chula had to be given special attention to help her get over her outrage at the new addition to life at the rancho. Nata finally emerged from puppyhood, and in time the two dogs made their peace. They would hunt together, and Nata joined Chula as companion and guardian for Joaquin during times she was alone, both dogs sleeping in her hermitage every night. It was many months before

Sister Joaquin could find an extra hour even to take a mid-day siesta before the people started coming to the clinic. She complained that her time for prayer and reading seemed to her to have become an "illusion," given the demands of her immediate world.[6]

Sister Jane accompanied Joaquin to Santa Fe on one of the trips to get papers revalidated, and the two planned to return to Mexico the next day. They were staying at Santa Fe's Immaculate Heart of Mary Seminary, and as they were leaving, Jane missed a step: "I flew across that porch and cracked my hip," Jane wrote to the Sisters in Ohio. "You could hear it all over—and my head missed an iron pole by about five inches, or I would have been crushed in the head. I really hit hard. She [Joaquin] just about died. She said, 'stay there.' I said, 'Honey, I couldn't move if I tried.' Jane was rushed by ambulance to St. Vincent's. Joaquin stayed with her for two days, but then returned to Mexico, once again without the friend she had wished to work with her for so long.[7]

Once the legal problems with Father Aelred's will were worked out, the monastery of Christ in the Desert took control of the 33-acre property at Rancho de la Soledad. Prior Philip had promised the dying Father Aelred that the land would become a Benedictine monastery. However, the community at the New Mexico monastery was too small to establish a formal monastic foundation in Mexico. The Chama brothers tried to give the property away to other Benedictine monasteries, but there were no takers. They soon realized that they would have to keep it themselves and develop the monastery that Aelred had dreamed of, and continue his work with the villagers. Brother Christopher and Brother Francisco, in addition to helping to finish the school, working on the well project and the bridge and helping the workers market their crafts, set about remodeling the existing buildings with the hope that in time Mexican monks would come and a formal monastery could be established. They maintained the Benedictine ritual of the Divine Office as had Father Aelred. The change in ownership required a survey of the land. The survey showed one side of the property was bordered by the historic road along which Padre Miguel Hidalgo y Costilla and his army had carried the flag of Mexico between

Atotonilco and Dolores Hidalgo in his failed 1810 call for independence from Spain. The survey also showed the land was about two acres less than Fr. Aelred had been told he had bought— to the advantage of their neighbor. There was no point in discussing this—better to let it go. It was more important to keep good relations in the neighborhood.

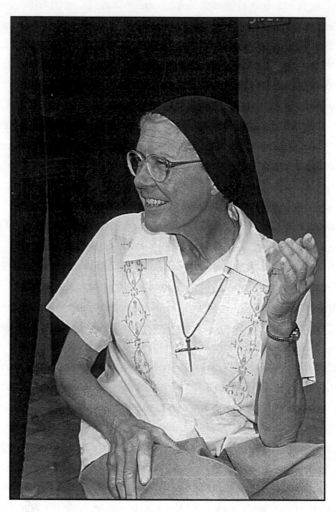

Sister Mary Joaquin, La Soledad, 1987.
Photograph: Deborah Douglas collection.

In1987, two monks from the Abbey of Tepeyac, Father Ezequiel Bas Luna and Brother Fernando Hool Salazar, joined Sister Joaquin and the two brothers from New Mexico to help with the work. Brother Fernando is an architect, which made their construction efforts much easier. The two Mexican monks were the first to permanently settle in what would ultimately become the Monasterio Nuestra Señora de la Soledad. Gradually, with much work over the years by the brothers and helped later by Sister Joaquin's fundraising campaign, the monastery was completed in 1994.

11

~†~

*I*n July 1988, Sister Joaquin's dear friend and personal doctor, Bergere Kenney, died. For years Joaquin had worked closely with Dr. Kenney as the head of her medical staff at St. Vincent Hospital, and in 1968 as the first chairman of the hospital's new community Board of Trustees. Driving up from Mexico to Santa Fe for the funeral, she listened to Mahler's great *Resurrection Symphony* on a tape in her car. At the funeral, she described the feelings for her friend that the music had elicited in her. "The music is powerful, and so was the life of Bergere Kenney, touching so many lives, advising, counseling, healing—a word of wisdom here, a word of encouragement there—always selfless, with a certain charm and humility, always open to our needs." She went on to describe an incident at St. Vincent's that she felt would give an understanding of the doctor's nature:

> He called my office one day to ask if I could come to the delivery room right away. I hurried up the back stairs wondering what great emergency was awaiting me, only to find Bergere looking out the window with a pair of field glasses at a mother hawk and her chicks in the weeping willow tree.... Bergere was no ordinary man; he was very special. We have no reason to feel any sorrow for him, only for ourselves for having lost him.[1]

For Mary Joaquin, the death of Bergere Kenney brought not only grief at the loss of a great friend and former colleague. She had also lost the doctor who had treated her incurable illness for the past twenty years, and who had helped provide her with medical supplies for her Mexico clinic.

In September, Joaquin decided to make a trip back to the Motherhouse in Cincinnati and visit her family in Wapakoneta. She was very close to her sister and her nephews and nieces. Sister Jane, who frequently visited Joaquin's family with her, recalled later that there was always music playing in the house, along with the smell of delicious, fresh-baked Italian cookies.

But travel was becoming more and more difficult for Joaquin. Her arthritic condition and the Raynaud's disease were progressing. Her X-rays showed a complete loss of cartilage in her right shoulder, with bone painfully rubbing on bone, making driving extremely painful. Within two weeks of her return to Mexico, she came to the decision that she could no longer continue her work there. Her mission at La Soledad was ended; it was time to return to her own country.

Father Ezequiel wrote that the villagers wailed when they heard the news: "And now what will we do without Madrecita?"[2] The villagers and monks threw her a lavish *despedida*—a bittersweet goodbye party.

Although Mary Joaquin's Spanish was still very elementary, Father Ezequiel recalled that the people understood her and she them because she spoke to them and listened to them with such love. Sometimes it was a tough love, as when she scolded the women for giving their babies what she believed was *pulque*, a traditional alcoholic drink from fermented maguey juice. The women explained that what they were giving was the *aqua miel*, or "honey water," before the juice ferments into *pulque*, and which they insisted built up the baby's strength and "thickened the blood." Joaquin was not convinced—she worried that the *agua miel* would give the child a predisposition to alcoholism, and alcoholism was only too prevalent in the village. But the people loved her and knew that her scoldings were out of concern for them. If a child needed a shot, there was always candy to help overcome the tears. She provided the very poor with clothes and bought shoes for them. At Christmas she always had a party for the children with candy and piñatas.

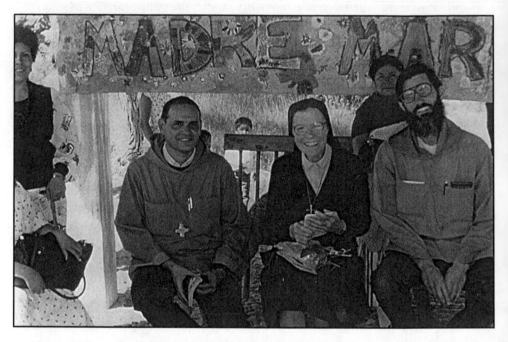

Farewell Party for Sister Mary Joaquin ("Madre Maria"). La Soledad, 1988. Photograph: Benigno Baltazar family

Sister Joaquin wrote to the friends who had donated money and materials for her clinic to tell them that she would be leaving La Soledad, and to urge them to continue their support. Donations could be made to her account at the Sunwest Bank in Santa Fe. In her letter she submitted her last annual report for September 1, 1987 to August 31, 1988. She had gained $12,200 in donations, a considerable sum for Mexico, and had spent $12,296:

Milk: $1539
Food: $635
Medicines: $5286
Hospital: $806
Other: $1410

"Other" included laboratory and X-ray charges, transportation, and 250 pairs of shoes. She counted 2126 sick visits for the year, with the same diseases that she had encountered the decade before: amoebic dysentery, respiratory infections, diarrhea associated with malnutrition, eye and ear infections.[3] During the twelve years of her mission at La Soledad, she counted over 16,000 sick visits.

The future of the clinic was unsure. Brother Francisco agreed to help out for a short while, but he had much work to do at La Soledad and his ministry to the villagers. The two monks at La Soledad were hoping that another religious group would send help to the rancho to continue Sister Joaquin's work. A group of Mexican Benedictine nuns from La Catequista de Maria Santissima in Querétero did take over the clinic for a time, dispensing bandages and certain medicines, but the nuns were not nurses, and soon the clinic closed. Christ in the Desert maintained a medical fund to help some of the worst cases in Los Rico. There were two doctors and a dentist in San Miguel who provided free care. Mary Joaquin had sent her patients to them, and she would pay for the medicines. The monks continued to help in this way, giving a needy patient a permit for the free help, and paying for the medicine.

Mary Joaquin was extremely disappointed that the clinic could not continue. Undoubtedly she had saved many lives in the twelve years she was at La Soledad—especially the lives of the malnourished babies and children who certainly would have died had she not been there to help them. But she had hoped to be able to start something that would survive without her. Although the clinic had to be closed, she was still especially concerned that the food program continue. She wrote to Prior Philip to urge his ongoing support, explaining how important the program was:

In 1977, when I went to La Soledad, I was shocked at the condition of the babies and children. Potbellies, stringy arms and legs and dull minds—all manifestations of malnutrition. It was a joy to see the children blossom after just a year of consistent food supplement. That word "consistent" is what's important... it's got to be regular. Sure, the men work (sometimes) and often had money, but the poor wives saw little of the money. All but about four or five men in Los Rico drank up the money, so the children didn't benefit at all.[4]

With the help of the Mexican nuns who distributed the food, the program did continue for another fifteen years, still funded by the Florida parishioners with help from Christ in the Desert and from friends in San Miguel. But that program finally ended as well.[5]

Joaquin was resigned—she had no choice. Her illness made continuing at La Soledad impossible for her. She told a reporter, "I used to plan this or that. "Now I just let it happen. That's following God's will, doing what the good Lord seems to tell you to do. The only thing is, He seems to put me someplace and then yank me out again. I can't quite figure that out."[6]

Sister Mary Joaquin's yearning for the contemplative life was still strong in her. Prior to leaving La Soledad, she had already determined to join the Carmelite monastery in Santa Fe, where a group of cloistered nuns spend their days in the isolation of a simple and prayerful life. After a lifetime of service, both as a nurse and administrator in American hospitals and as the only heath care provider for the *campesinos* of Los Rico, she was ready to withdraw to the convent world of quiet and prayer she had wanted for so many years. At the convent she would only be able to receive visitors every two months, although she could continue to write and receive mail. Her decision also meant to her that she should rid herself of all the letters and papers of her past life. Before she left the little Mexican hermitage that had been her home for twelve years, she built a huge bonfire in an oil drum and burned up a lifetime of correspondence.

The last to go in this "bonfire of the vanities," as a friend described it, was her Registered Nurse license. On November 17, 1988, Sister Mary Joaquin left La Soledad.[7]

Joaquin's decision to join the Carmelites meant that she could no longer be a member of the Sisters of Charity. The Carmelites are a different Order, and she would have to petition Rome for an indult to be allowed to change her affiliation.[8] She also had to petition the Cincinnati Sisters to allow her to transfer her vows to another Order. On October 26, 1988 she wrote to the Sisters:

> I want to thank you and all my sisters in our community for the blessed and grace-filled forty-five years I have spent as a Sister of Charity.... Each of us has a call from God to [serve] Him in the way He directs us. My years as a Sister of Charity prepared me well as I take yet another step in the service of our Lord Jesus Christ. I carry each one of you with me in love and prayer as I enter into the Monastery of Carmel of Santa Fe. I shall never forget you. Pray for me as I, too, shall be praying for you.[9]

The Executive Council of the Cincinnati Order approved the transfer. On November 22, 1988, sixteen Sisters of Charity living in New Mexico, along with many Santa Fe friends and monks from Christ in the Desert and La Soledad gathered for a "send off" for Sister Joaquin. Present from the Motherhouse was the elderly Sister Jean Clare Kenney, the sister who had encouraged the young student nurse, Gina Bitler, to join the Sisters of Charity in 1943. On December 8, without waiting for the indult from Rome, Sister Mary Joaquin disappeared behind the walls of the Santa Fe Monastery of Carmel.

By changing Orders, Mary Joaquin had to "begin again" as a new nun with the Carmelites. After a brief postulancy, she would make a novitiate for one or two years. She would live in temporary vows for three years before making Solemn Profession. After this long period of discernment, she would become a permanent member of the Order.

As a Carmelite nun, Joaquin was also required to take a new religious name. She chose the name Sister Mary Benedicta of the Cross, a decision that greatly pleased her friend from the Cincinnati Motherhouse, Sister Benedicta Mahoney, who had worried Gina would take that name back in 1943 before Benedicta could take it for herself.

But perhaps, in following her own strong desire, Sister Joaquin had misinterpreted God's will. She lasted at the Santa Fe convent for a little over two months. Sister Maryanna Cole, the new president of the Sisters of Charity, received a phone call from the new Carmelite postulant Mary Benedicta, telling the president that she had to leave the convent. The Carmelite nuns live an extremely austere life, refusing to use heat in their rooms. They gave Mary Benedicta extra blankets, and perhaps compromised their principles just a bit by giving her a space heater. They gave her work in the bakery because it was the warmest place in the convent. As a matter of occupancy requirements, the Santa Fe City building code required that the convent must have heat. But the nuns never turned it on. "I would look at that Honeywell dial on the wall, but I couldn't bring myself to touch it," Sister Joaquin said later to friends. "It was against the rules of the convent."[10]

Mary Benedicta's illness in the cold of Santa Fe's winter grew worse, becoming so extreme that the nuns feared her toes might have to be amputated. She was rushed to St. Vincent Hospital, where twelve years earlier she had stopped at the door, saying that her work there was finished. Her toes recovered, but her time with the Carmelites was ended. It was a profound disappointment for her, since the cloistered convent had seemed the answer to her perennial search for the contemplative life. The Sisters of Charity welcomed Sister Mary Joaquin back to the Motherhouse as one of their own.

Part III

≈†≈

Christ in the Desert. Abiquiú, New Mexico

> The liturgy was simple but
> beautiful, as only the Benedictines
> can do it…. There was a deep
> feeling of universality present.
> —Sister Mary Joaquin

12

~†~

*I*n Cincinnati, the doctors realized that the sudden deterioration of Mary Joaquin's condition while with the Carmelites was caused by an imbalance in the medications she was taking. When this was corrected, Joaquin's physical condition improved. But she had slid into a state of profound despondency. She was angry with God. In her heart she could not accept the loss of her dream of entering the Carmel cloister. For some weeks at the Motherhouse she was profoundly depressed. "It was my dark night of the soul," she told friends later, referring to John of the Cross's description of his struggle to reconcile God's will over his own deep desires. "Then one day," Joaquin related. "as I was sitting at breakfast with the sisters, one of them said something very funny, and I burst out laughing. I suddenly realized that my laughter that morning was the beginning of the end of my 'dark night.'"[1] She was soon well again in her mind, and sufficiently recovered in her body that she was eager to leave the Motherhouse. She wrote to Prior Philip at Christ in the Desert:

> By looking back on leaving La Soledad and entering Carmel, I really was angry at God for seemingly leading me down the rose-strewn path only to take me out and drag me—nowhere! When I realized through the gift of faith, that all this was God's

loving plan for me, and that He was still loving and leading me, then the depression lifted, prayer returned, and my whole body began to improve.[2]

In her recovery, Joaquin felt so well in body and mind that she considered returning to La Soledad. Not only was she concerned about the needs of the poor of Los Rico, she would also be able to return to the eremitic life she had established for herself there. Prior Philip advised her against this. He felt that she might soon have to leave again, and it was better to let the people at La Soledad and Los Rico come up with their own solutions to the problems there.

If she could not be a cloistered nun in Santa Fe or a monastic in Mexico, Joaquin still was determined to return to a hermit's life. She knew she couldn't find the quiet and peace she still so profoundly desired in the bustle of activity at the Motherhouse. She asked Prior Philip if she could live at Christ in the Desert. She remembered there was a primitive little house at the edge of the Chama River on the monastery property that had once housed a family in the 1960s. It could be the hermitage she was seeking. Even though she was aware the winters of northern New Mexico could be snowy and cold—in fact she had already suffered that cold during visits to the monastery—she was willing to risk the weather. The prior invited her to come and join the brothers in New Mexico.

Some of the Cincinnati sisters couldn't understand Joaquin's desire to leave the Motherhouse, and were baffled by her intense need for solitude. She wrote them a long letter to try to explain what her experiences in Mexico had meant to her, and why she was drawn to continue the quiet life she had experienced there. Despite the hassles of well-drilling and bridge building and driving the sick to the doctor and spending afternoons running her clinic, there were indeed -periods of the day when she was able to experience a time of deep prayer in which she could achieve a quiet, transcendent communion with God. Her letter was later published as an article in the Sisters of Charity magazine, *Intercom*:

The ring of the alarm clock awakened me at 3 am for the start of a new day. I quickly dressed by candlelight. As I walked to the chapel, the stars surrounded me like a cloak, calming my mind and spirit in preparation for the first Hour of the Divine Office, Vigils. By kerosene lamps we chanted the psalms and listened to the readings from the Fathers of the Church. It was still dark when I returned to my hermitage, and the stars, like so many nations and peoples of the world surrounded me with their closeness…. [There was] complete silence, such that I could hear the swish of the birds' wings as they flew over.

It is in utter silence that the self with all its weaknesses looms large, until one day self diminishes and God encompasses all. It is in the love of God that one meets all peoples of the world. It is in this silence that one shares in the sufferings, oppressions and heartaches of our brothers and sisters everywhere. The more one loses oneself in God, the more one becomes united with all creation. In the words of John of the Cross, "at the summit of prayer we experience creatures through the Creator."

The chanting of the seven Hours of the Divine Office, spaced as they are throughout the day, kept my mind and body anchored in God as necessary duties and work were performed. The washing clothes by hand, smelling their freshness as I hung them up to dry, was another touch of God's nearness. Cooking simple, meatless meals brought the poor closer. Experiencing living without "things" as the poor do makes externals and material things fade into oblivion and you know how unimportant they are.

Early morning before Vigils was my favorite time for prayer. The silence is deafening, not even a donkey braying or a rooster crowing. Then for Mass there was celebration and singing. Twenty or more people joined us for the Eucharist and over a hundred on Sundays, forming one close family. My day ended as it had begun, praising God at Compline and thanking Him for the day.[3]

In late 1989, Sister Joaquin left Cincinnati to return to New Mexico, to the little hermitage at the edge of the Chama River. It was located a considerable distance from the main activity of the monastery chapel and refectory and from the many visitors to the monastery's guesthouse. The hermitage was a simple ten-by-ten room with a wood stove, a writing desk, a bed, a wooden rocker, and a shelf for her books. There was no electricity or cook stove; she would take her meals in the refectory with the monks. She brought her treasured icon from Greece and other religious pictures to adorn the walls. Outside, she had a small wooden bench where she could sit and watch the river and the orange sandstone cliffs opposite. The quiet, almost silent flow of the river made the little bench a place for prayer and meditation. It was too far for her to walk to the chapel to celebrate the Hours of the Divine Office, but she could drive to the chapel along the often-muddy monastery dirt road. She kept to the Benedictine schedule as she had at La Soledad, arriving at 4 am mornings for Vigils in the chapel with the brothers. Nights could be cold and difficult for her, but the brothers kept her well provided with split logs for her wood stove, and they gave her a gas heater. Once in a while she would drive into Santa Fe, two hours to the south, to see friends or meet with her doctor, occasionally to Mexico to visit La Soledad and her Los Rico friends. She still wrote to the donors who had given to the clinic and the food program, asking them to continue helping the people at La Soledad.

Christmas at her monastery home was a moving celebration for Joaquin. She related her experience of Christmas in the desert in a letter to a friend at the Motherhouse:

On my way to Christmas Vigils at 10:30 pm the stars were so bright it was unbelievable. Then as I drew near the chapel, it seemed suspended in the cold clear mountain air. The monks and guests had put out hundreds of *farolitos*; there was no wind so they flickered in their little sacks and seemed to tell me Jesus is coming! Jesus is here! The liturgy was simple but beautiful, as only the Benedictines can do it. At the Offertory, the three Vietnamese monks sang a beautiful oriental hymn to Mary, accompanied by bells and stringed instruments, and at the prayers of the faithful, each nationality prayed for world peace in his own language. There was a deep feeling of universality present.[4]

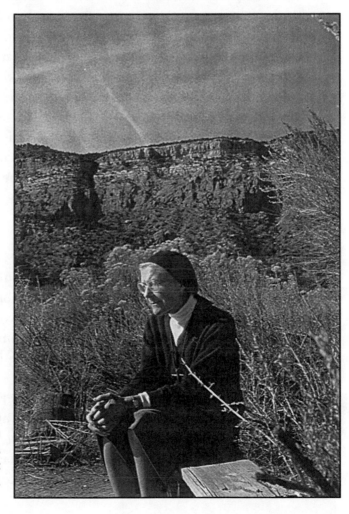

Sister Mary Joaquin at her hermitage on the Chama River. Photograph: Jennifer Levy.

For the next two years, Joaquin lived the life of contemplative prayer that she had so devoutly wished for. She had as much solitude as she felt she needed on a daily basis, and also she could maintain her contacts in Santa Fe. The Santa Fe community had not forgotten her, even if most people, outside of her friends, probably hadn't seen her for the last fourteen years. During those years, the newspapers kept her name before the public, publishing articles on her work in Mexico with the clinic and the food program, as well as with the well project. In December 1990, St. Vincent Hospital celebrated its 125 years in Santa Fe with the groundbreaking for the new $4 million Emergency Room and Cancer Treatment Center wings. Sister Joaquin was on hand to help celebrate. It was a Christmas party and the whole town was invited with enough cake and punch for 2000 people. Santa Claus was there as well, holding the children on his knee and listening to their wishes. Joaquin joked that Santa Claus was a hard act to follow. She gave a brief history of the Sisters of Charity's role in establishing Santa Fe's first and still-only hospital: "They suffered some," she said, "but served many. They planted and watered the seed that was to bear such magnificent fruit." The only downside to the celebration was that the weather prevented the planned hot air balloon rides.[5]

∼†∼

The buildings of Christ in the Desert were built in the 1960s, and some of them were in sad need of repair. The monastery had grown, and not only repairs were necessary, but new accommodations and a larger refectory were needed for the increasing number of monks. One early snowing morning, Brother Bernard, coming from his cell on his way to early morning Vigils in the dark, fell on the ice and broke his leg. The accident convinced the monks that something had to be done soon to improve their living conditions. Furthermore, this was the time that money was needed to continue the work building the new foundation at La Soledad. The brothers developed an extensive plan for repairs and for new buildings. They calculated they would need to raise three million dollars—a sum, as it later turned out, that grossly underestimated the cost of their ambitious plans. In honor of their founder, they initiated the Father Aelred Wall Memorial Campaign to raise funds for the work. And who better to chair the campaign and twist arms for such a worthy cause than the woman, well known to the Santa Fe public, who had been so successful fundraising for the hospital and for her clinic? So Sister Mary Joaquin's quiet life changed, caught up once again in the "external" world.

The brothers put together a national campaign committee of nineteen members that included the names of the rich and famous—Hollywood celebrities, well-known artists and writers, prominent Church officials. Father Aelred's sister was among the members, as was the writer Tony Hillerman, the actress, Loretta Young, Bob Hope's wife Dolores, the Bishop of Celaya, the Archbishop of Santa Fe, and the daughter of architect Nakashima, the man who had built the chapels at Christ in the Desert and La Soledad for Father Aelred. The honorary chairperson was the film and stage actress, Jane Wyatt, who had been a friend of Father Aelred. The kick-off event was held on July 25, 1991 at the El Dorado Hotel in Santa Fe in honor of Sister Mary Joaquin, with Jane Wyatt as the guest of honor.

With her new position as chair of the Aelred Wall Memorial Campaign Sister Joaquin was again in the news. The lunch in her honor at the El Dorado Hotel gave Governor Bruce King the opportunity to issue a Proclamation:

> *I hereby proclaim July 25, 1991 as "'Sister Mary Joaquin Bitler Day" in New Mexico, and invite the people of New Mexico to participate in the day's ceremonies, and express thanks and appreciation for Sister Mary Joaquin's dedicated and faithful service to the people of New Mexico and the world."*

Not to be outdone by the governor, Santa Fe Mayor Sam Pick proclaimed "Sister Mary Joaquin Day" for the city as well in a formal *Bando Official de la Villa Real de Santa Fé de San Francisco de Asis.*

At the luncheon, among talks by several friends and dignitaries, Seth Montgomery, her good friend and the lawyer who had presided over St. Vincent Hospital's many legal issues, described the hours Sister Joaquin had spent working to get the new St. Vincent Hospital built:

> There were probably thousands of hours spent by Sister as chief planner, chief construction superintendent, chief architect, chief financial consultant, chief negotiator, chief hospital administrator—and yes, chief legal strategist. [I]t required an extraordinary blend of talents: lobbying city and county governments, the state legislature, and the federal Hill-Burton agency to name a few; working with contractors, architects, hospital consultants and health care professionals; managing and directing lawyers, accountants, investment bankers, land use planners, and many, many others. It was a heady experience in high finance, business planning, and hospital management. And when it was all over, Sister withdrew from the scene and went to work as a hermit nun in a lonely village in the high desert of central Mexico.[6]

The luncheon organizers, Peggy Jones and Mimi Woodbridge, were delighted that the luncheon event brought in $12,000 for the two monasteries.

For the next five years, Sister Joaquin and her committee managed the local fundraising, while others took on the national effort. In keeping with the Benedictine tradition of open hospitality, the guesthouse at Christ in the Desert had welcomed distinguished visitors from all over the country and even abroad, and many of these were solicited to help in the fundraising effort. Joaquin was rather appalled at the task expected of her, and asked her friend Lew Thompson to help her. Lew owned the public relations firm she had hired in the 1970s to handle public relations issues for Saint Vincent Hospital.

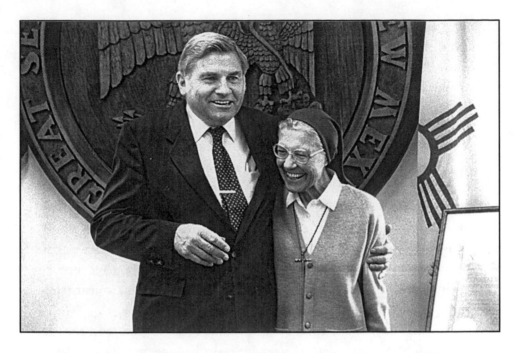

Governor Bruce King proclaims July 25, 1991 "Sister Mary Joaquin Bitler Day."
Photograph: Monastery of Christ in the Desert Archives

The two of them and their committee organized fund-raising dinners and auctions. With the assistance of Santa Fe gallery owners and the Thomas Merton Study Center in Louisville, Kentucky, they arranged for a show and sale of copies of Thomas Merton's photographs. Shortly before Merton was accidentally killed on a trip to Bangkok in 1968, he had twice stayed at Christ in the Desert. He had even considered Christ in the Desert as a possible venue for an East-West center that would be a forum for international peace. His trip to Asia had been with the intent to explore the possibility of such a center with Buddhist leaders. Merton was an excellent photographer, and had made photographs of the monastery, of Georgia O'Keefe, and of the desert plants and landscape. The show and sale was to commemorate the twenty-five years since Merton's death.

On another occasion, fifty artists were invited by the committee to spend time at the monastery to paint, draw, or sculpt their impressions of the landscape; the art was then sold at a fundraiser in Santa Fe. The campaign applied for grants, and the first received was $100,000 from a Chicago foundation, which the brothers used to renovate their chapel; they insulated the roof, fixed cracked trusses, and installed thermal glass in the clerestory windows.

Over the next few years, with the help from the fundraisers, the monastery at La Soledad was brought to completion, and Christ in the Desert built a cloister of cells for the monks and a new refectory and gift shop. The construction at the Chama monastery became an award winning world model for the use of sustainable resources—the use of straw bales as construction material and wood from sustainable forests, a field of solar panels to light and heat the buildings, and a constructed wetlands to process the monastery's waste water.[7]

Sister Joaquin drove frequently to Santa Fe for committee meetings and fundraiser lunches and dinners. It must have seemed to her like a repeat of her past life of the 1960s when she was desperately struggling to raise enough money to keep St. Vincent Hospital's doors open. Her friends were concerned that after some of these events she would have to drive back to the monastery in the dark, and they were especially worried about her driving at night along the last thirteen miles of two-rut dirt road that curls along the sides of the cliffs above the river. The management of the Inn of the Governors generously offered Joaquin a room for the night whenever it got too late for her to safely return home, and if the manager expected the Inn to be full, friends would pay to reserve a room for her.

However, it was not only the night driving that was dangerous. By the mid-1990s, the fundraising had allowed the monastery to start construction, and heavy trucks were making deep ruts in the muddy road. Sister Joaquin knew she needed a better car, one that had high enough clearance not to drag on the road. She wrote to Sister Grace Ann in Cincinnati for permission to buy a new car:

I drove out the thirteen miles (from the monastery to the highway) and it took me one hour and ten minutes. The road was very muddy and slippery and I came close to slipping off the road twice. There's a 60-foot drop down to the Chama River. My car scrapes bottom, and I had a $500 repair job when I got to town. The same thing happened last week.... I came very near the edge of the road and by the time I reached the highway I was a nervous wreck. I spend $250 a month on my car. I would adjust my budget some way to make that $350 a month.[8]

At La Soledad, Mary Joaquin had adored her dog Nata, but, alas, Nata had to be left behind in Mexico. Friends gave Mary Joaquin a puppy to be her companion at the little Chama hermitage. Once again she was confronted with dog training, this time requiring trips into town to Bruno's trainer, scheduled to coincide with fundraising committee meetings and doctor appointments. Always the dog lover, Joaquin was delighted to have the little pup sleeping at the foot of her bed every night. But Bruno did not survive his puppyhood. He got out of his fenced area and was found drowned at the edge of the river, leaving behind a grieving Sister Joaquin.

During the years of the fundraising activities, Mary Joaquin's health continued to deteriorate. She made a quick trip back to the Motherhouse in 1993 with Prior Philip to celebrate her fiftieth year as a Sister of Charity, but such long-distance travel was difficult for her. The rheumatoid arthritis had not only attacked her bones, but also her endocrine glands. The connective tissue disease was now affecting her joints, as well as her intestines and esophagus, causing burning and difficulty swallowing. The scleraderma had spread all over her body, making her skin extremely dry; it and would crack without use of a prescription lotion. Dr. Weiner, the Santa Fe orthopedist, told her that the disease in one of her hip joints had become so serious that she must have a hip replacement. If she didn't have the surgery, the situation would only become worse.

The Sisters of Charity wanted Joaquin to come back to Cincinnati to have the surgery in the hospital there. Joaquin wrote to Sister John Miriam, strongly arguing against returning to the Motherhouse, saying that she wanted to have the operation with the doctors who knew her, and who had followed the progress of her disease over the years, seeing her every three to four months. She assured Sister John that she felt "peaceful and calm" about the procedure. While Dr. Weiner performed the surgery, Drs. Suhre and La Farge would be in the operating room to monitor her heartbeat and circulation, and would put a pacer in if her heartbeat became too slow. "I know practically everyone in that hospital [St. Vincent's]," she wrote, " and it feels 'like home.'" As an obedient, if stubborn, nun, she of course told Sister John: "After considering all things, you still want me to come to Cincy, I would, of course, obey." But she added, "I would be less than truthful if I didn't say, however, that if I have to go to Cincy, I'd be very uptight and scared.... I want to do God's will in this and am praying for light and direction. But I feel it is necessary to present my side, so a proper decision can be made. After all, it is my body."[9]

The Sisters acquiesced, and the operation was performed at St. Vincent's. Joaquin spent three weeks recovering in the home of two Sisters of Our Lady of the Desert in Española, both of whom were nurses. She returned to the monastery after a month, and two weeks later she was able to drive again.

Because of her deteriorating health, it was becoming difficult for Joaquin to stay in the little hermitage by the river, and she was spending more and more nights at the Inn of the Governors in Santa Fe. Additionally, the brothers were concerned that the hermitage, so close to the riverbank, might one day be carried away in a flood. They felt it should be torn down. With the first of the new buildings at Christ in the Desert almost finished, the noted New Mexico writer Tony Hillerman and his wife, Maria, funded the construction of two additional infirmary cells at the monastery, one of which was intended for Mary Joaquin. She moved into a comfortable, radiant-heated room. The other cell was occasionally occupied by a visiting sister from the Motherhouse, sometimes by her friend Marguerite, and once by her blood sister, Frances Herbst from

Ohio, who came for an extended stay with her. It wasn't the remote and charming hermitage by the river that she indeed preferred, but for the first time since leaving the Motherhouse, Sister Joaquin could live her contemplative vocation in a comfortable, warm room.

13

~†~

*I*n 1996, Sister Joaquin's close friend Marguerite Claffey was in St. Vincent Hospital for throat surgery. Joaquin would come to Santa Fe from Christ in the Desert to visit her. As well as offering Marguerite support and condolence, the visits offered Joaquin the opportunity—an opportunity not available to her at the monastery—to watch the sports channel on the hospital room television. An avid Tiger Woods fan, Joaquin joined Marguerite's son Tom in his mother's hospital room so together they could watch Tiger Woods at the Masters.

But the next year's visit to St. Vincent's was not for TV sports entertainment. Tom and Mary Joaquin were at Marguerite's bedside to comfort her as she was dying. Father Leo Lucero from Cristo Rey Church came to give Marguerite the last rites. After his mother's death, Tom visited one of the local priests to discuss arrangements for the funeral Mass. He mentioned that Marguerite's wish was that her ashes be scattered above the little grotto to Our Lady of Lourdes near the village of Los Ojos in northern New Mexico. The priest said absolutely not. The grotto had never been consecrated. Catholic ashes could not be scattered, could only be buried in a container in consecrated ground, and then only with the permission of the local parish priest. Sister Joaquin's quiet, straightforward response when she heard this was, "Tom, I feel you and I should carry out your mother's wishes just as she stated them."

The following April, Joaquin joined Tom and his wife Silvia, and the three of them drove north to the grotto. It had been snowing and the ground was rough, but the two helped Joaquin down to the grotto to celebrate their own private memorial. They had asked no one else to join them. They scattered Marguerite's ashes at the grotto as she had wanted, returning her to the Chama Valley where she began her life. There was no priest present and none had been consulted. Tom knew he needed no higher authority from the Catholic Church than Sister Mary Joaquin.[1]

Marguerite's estate was not large, but in her will, she stated: "To my dearly beloved friend … the sum of $5000." Because of her vow of poverty, Sister Joaquin could not accept such a gift, even though her medical expenses were considerable. Tom, who considered Joaquin as his older sister—she was only twelve years older than he—solved her problem by dispensing the money to her as needed for her "maintenance."

Certainly, Sister Joaquin was an obedient nun. Her vow of poverty prevented her from accepting a monetary gift. But regarding Church regulations that hindered her doing what she believed in her heart was "right"—whether providing birth control injections that hinder a baby from being born only to inhabit a coffin, or carrying out the last request of a dying friend—she made her own decisions

Scleraderma means "hard skin." By the end of 1999, the scleraderma had spread to many parts of Joaquin's body, and she constantly needed to apply a special prescription lotion on her skin. Besides the ulcers on her fingertips and toes, the collagen material from the scleraderma had invaded her intestines, a portion of her heart, her esophagus and her stomach. As well as creating painful, physical problems for her—it was difficult for her to swallow—the disease was creating financial problems as well. She wrote to Sister Grace Ann at the Motherhouse, explaining that the cost of her medicines would mean that she needed an additional $500 a month, and that she knew that would take her over the Order's budget limit for sisters living independently. She listed the cost of each medical item in great detail. She was clearly embarrassed to ask for the money, "I have never gone this high on my budget, never."[2] Five years earlier, she had argued strongly against leaving New Mexico and returning to Cincinnati for her hip operation. Undoubtedly she feared that her request for more money would trigger the call to "come home" to the Motherhouse, a call that she stubbornly would not wish to obey. It did not. However, the next year she wrote again to Sister Grace Ann that she planned to leave Christ in the Desert and return to Cincinnati in two years. She asked that a room be reserved for her. She was seventy-eight and sick; she knew it would be her final move.

But her final move came sooner than she had planned. A little over a year after she wrote the letter to Sister Grace Ann, she was back in St. Vincent Hospital. This time the brothers felt she was too sick to return to living at the monastery, where medical help was a great distance away. In the hospital, she had already come to this decision herself; it was time to go to the Motherhouse. In March 2001, she went back to the monastery only to gather her few possessions and return to the Inn of the Governors, where Sister Pat Bernard found her extremely ill, and accompanied her back on an airplane to Cincinnati.

Joaquin moved into the Motherhouse assisted living quarters, Mother Margaret Hall. From her window she could see the little chapel where she had once made her vows to the Sisters of Charity almost fifty-eight years earlier. The move had been a difficult, if necessary, decision for her. She still struggled with accepting the inevitable, much as she had struggled against other forced moves in her life. Perhaps the struggle was with her own disappointment—the anger at her weakening condition, the conflict of subordinating her own desires to the inevitability of accepting God's will. She had wanted to die in her own way, not in the Motherhouse hospital. Her friend Sister Jane later said: "Joaquin really wanted to die in Mexico."[3]

The sisters helped Joaquin in her struggle, offering her their counseling and prayers. Her friends sent her music tapes that she played constantly in her room. Sister Jane commented that when she went to Mother Margaret Hall to visit her, Joaquin would be lying in bed in pain, but would sit up immediately her friend entered with a bright, welcoming smile as if nothing were wrong. But as she was leaving, Jane would glance back and see Joaquin curled back in pain in the fetal position.

Sister Joaquin lingered on at Mother Margaret Hall for another two and a half years, her scleraderma and the Raynaud's phenomenon becoming progressively worse. Her friends would call her from Santa Fe and send her gifts; some came to Cincinnati to visit her. But as she neared death, she could no longer talk to them. Just before she died, her friend Lew Thompson called her. The sisters told him she was no longer able to speak, but she could listen to him. So Lew talked to her for an hour on the phone in a one-sided conversation. The nuns told him the call had made her very happy. Sister Joaquin died later that day, on May, 26, 2003, three days after her eighty-first birthday, and almost sixty years after joining the Sisters of Charity.

Several friends came from Santa Fe for her funeral at the Motherhouse. Sister Joaquin had been Deborah Douglas's spiritual director, and Deborah gave a talk to the assembled mourners, explaining how "Madre," as she always called her, had encouraged her in her spiritual life, and how Joaquin had inspired her husband David to start his "Waterlines" business after his experience with the Los Rico well. "Madre sought always to find and to do the will of God," Deborah said, " to participate in Christ's love for the poor to the absolute limits of her strength, to trust in God's purposes even in the darkest times."

Sister Mary Joaquin Bitler, SC was buried on a hill above the Ohio River in the Sisters of Charity cemetery. She lies now in the company of the hundreds of nuns who have gone before her. Stored in the basement of the Motherhouse is the archive box containing the letters, newspaper clippings, and announcements of the many awards that recount the achievements of a remarkable life. There is only a single earthly possession in the box, the one Joaquin had kept with her to the end: the Hohner harmonica her Uncle Don had given her when she was ten years old.

Epilogue

~†~

S t. Vincent Hospital has remained the only general health care facility in Santa Fe, and more than once has fought off possible takeovers by for-profit HMOs. There was always concern in the community that if St. Vincent's became a for-profit hospital, there would be problems with maintaining indigent health care. The quarter-cent sales tax that Sister Mary Joaquin worked so hard to get passed in 1968 is today still providing indigent funds for the region. The only other full-service hospital in Santa Fe is the Indian Health Service facility, which provides hospital care to Native Americans from northern New Mexico.[1]

The hospital on St. Michael's Drive has gone through many changes and expansions to accommodate an increasing northern New Mexico population since it opened its doors in 1977. Of the many important changes was the opening in 1983 of the cancer center, and the 1985 a psychiatric center for adults and adolescents. And it has suffered some shocks: a 1980 prison riot that resulted in the sudden arrival by helicopter of 200 injured patients, most of them inmates, and a 10-day nurses' strike in 1988.

In 2007, after much local controversy, a group of investors won city development approval, and the private Physicians Medical Center opened in Santa Fe. There has been considerable concern in Congress regarding the economic impact of private specialty hospitals on general community hospitals, as well as potential ethical problems of doctors referring patients to a facility in which the doctors themselves have a financial interest.[2] The proposed Physician's Medical Center had been discussed since 2000, and is the first opened in Santa Fe aside from St. Vincent's and the Indian Health Service Hospital. Many residents as well as the administration of St. Vincent's had argued strongly against allowing private for-profit hospitals in the city, fearing they would attract some of the St. Vincent doctors, as well as siphon off paying patients, leaving the hospital with a greater debt for indigent care.[3] But the new Physicians Medical Center is small—only twelve beds—and is focused primarily on orthopedic surgery. It has, indeed, caused St. Vincent's to lose some of its doctors, but new ones come, and so far it appears not enough paying patients have been drawn away to cause a significant financial hardship.

In an ironic twist, after Sister Joaquin had planned so carefully to have the Sisters of Charity relinquish the Catholic St. Vincent's to nondenominational community ownership, forty years later, in 2008, St. Vincent Hospital merged with Christus Health, a Texas-based nonprofit Catholic hospital organization. The Santa Fe hospital has now been renamed the Christus-St. Vincent Regional Medical Center. And to further the irony, Christus Health was formed in 1999 by the merger of two Catholic health care systems, one of which was the Sisters of Charity Health Care System.[4]

With the Christus-St. Vincent merger, there was concern in the community, as well as by the state Human Services and Health Departments, as to the impact of Catholic ethical and religious directives on patient care. Of particular concern were the issues of family planning services, end-of-life choices, and the provision of reproductive services. To answer these concerns, a separate nonprofit, SVH SupportCo, was organized to provide services that conflict with Catholic directives.[5]

Christus Health maintains more than forty hospitals and other health care facilities in the United States and Mexico, with $4.1 billion in assets. Alex Valdez, CEO of St. Vincent's, emphasized that the infusion of $37 million that the partnership merger brings will remove all the hospital's existing debt and permit renovation and expansion of the facility, allowing for better patient care.[6] To date, the improved financial situation has permitted—among several upgrades—an expansion to five operating rooms beyond the single room in use since the hospital on St Michael's Drive opened, and a soon-to-be completed system of digitized medical records.[7]

~†~

Although Sister Joaquin's clinic closed after she left La Soledad in 1988, the *monasterio* at La Soledad still provides help to the villagers of Los Rico in emergency cases, giving passes for free doctor visits and paying for some medicines on a very limited basis. Four Benedictine sisters from the convent of Maria Santissima now live at La Soledad and, until it was ended a few years ago, distributed the food from the program that Mary Joaquin started. The sisters instruct the villagers in sanitation and proper nutrition and help the women with marketing goods they have made, such as children's clothes and various household articles.

Los Rico has changed considerably over the past few years. There is now electricity and running water in the houses throughout the village along with the ubiquitous cell phone and the occasional TV set. Some of the people now have cars or trucks and are able to drive to work or to a doctor or the hospital in San Miguel. They also can utilize the government clinic in Atotonilco some three miles away. If not for Sister Joaquin, many of these people would not have lived to adulthood. There have been some successes and some failures in her attempts to control the alcoholism. One of the worker's condition was so severe he would throw up blood when he drank. Today, thanks to Mary Joaquin, he is sober. Another, who would pass out for hours after imbibing sugar cane alcohol mixed with Coca Cola, now leads an AA group of about ten in Los Rico.[8]

The village well continues to produce an abundant flow of clean water twenty-four hours a day—a rarity in rural Mexico, where often water is available only three or four days a week. The suspension footbridge over the Laja River was twice damaged by floods, but has been repaired and is now far sturdier than before. Over the years the river cane the villagers planted to protect the bridge has spread and is holding the riverbank. Father Aelred's school was enlarged in 1990, with state teachers for kindergarten through the sixth grade. Also, the government has improved the road to the village, and more bus service has made it easier for the villagers to get to employment. Many of the women now work, mostly as hotel service workers or maids in private homes in San Miguel, and the families receive social welfare help from the government—as of 2009, approximately $35 per month for each child between ages six and seventeen. And as with many rural villages in Mexico, most families have a husband or uncle or son in the United States.

Today, the Monasterio Nuestra Señora de la Soledad has eleven monks, with Father Ezequiel as their superior. In 2004, they completed a large church that welcomes a hundred to two hundred people on a Sunday. Father Aelred's little chapel on the hill is still used for private meditation. The monastery is now self-sustaining, and welcomes pilgrims seeking a place of retreat. Sister Joaquin's little hermitage remains as it was when she lived there, and the picture of the woman she most admired, Mother Teresa of Calcutta, still hangs on the wall. The monks have come into the possession of a relic of Saint Benedict, a piece of bone, and several people claim to have been cured when Father Ezequiel places the relic on their forehead. However, a sign of modern times, unfortunately, is that the buildings at La Soledad must be kept locked to keep out thieves.

During her years as administrator of St Vincent Hospital, Sister Mary Joaquin performed her duties in conformance with the Sisters' mission of community service. She lived together with the other nuns at the convent in Marian Hall, and for a time was the superior of all the Sisters of Charity working locally. Her own high standards, her toughness, and her expectations concerning the performance of others made it perhaps inevitable that along with the many honors and awards given her by the Santa Fe community, she would also leave some enemies in her wake.

The 24/7 demands of effectively administering a major hospital took their toll in stress, and the legacy that has followed her years at the hospital is not without controversy. Not only was she physically suffering during much of that time, she was operating in a high-pressure managerial environment that was psychologically contrary to her profound desire to live a contemplative life. Undoubtedly such stress, if not precipitating her illness, certainly must have exacerbated the symptoms. And yet throughout those years, she hid the pain of her illness from her staff and her friends—most of whom remember only her open, captivating smile.

Perhaps it was from her engineer father that she inherited her disciplined strength of will to adhere to a rigorous daily schedule of solitude and prayer despite the distractions the world brought to her—the same strength that allowed her to be effective in a managerial position. And perhaps it was the influence of her artistic mother that nurtured her emotional nature, that allowed her to actively express love for those who were poor or suffering, but that also caused her to raise up her hands and rage at God for taking away her capacity to control them. Not only was the ability to play her beloved piano taken from her early on, in her later years her fingers on some days were incapable of even picking up a pencil. Both of these characteristics, the disciplined orderliness and the compassionate sensitivity, were combined in her nature. In some ways they complemented each other, and in some ways created great conflict in her. As her friend Brother Francisco from La Soledad pointed out:

> One of Sister Mary Joaquin's strongest assets was her strength of will and character over a long time of perseverance. It sometimes got in her way, but made possible much of what she accomplished in her apostolates and especially in her life of prayer and union with Christ, which must have been very difficult with her disease. She was known for her deep simplicity, and treated the very wealthy Americans and Mexicans in San Miguel Allende the same way she treated the poor people from Los Rico. They knew she was truly sincere and compassionate, especially with those who suffered.[9]

During Mary Joaquin's life as a Sister of Charity, the sisters were extremely patient with her independence—at times a stubborn independence. Certainly running a clinic for the poor is helping to fulfill the sisters' mission, but her longing for the *soledad* of a hermitage was contrary to the sisters' sense of community among themselves and the manner in which they carry out their social projects. Not that Joaquin didn't appreciate companionship, but only so far as it didn't interfere with her very private contemplative life. And when there was interference in that life, as there was many times at La Soledad and at Christ in the Desert—let alone the constant daily exigencies of hospital management— her letters show that the demands it made on her time for prayer and solitude were difficult for her to accept. Even in her fits of anger at God, she never lost her faith. In her prayers to discover God's intentions for her life, she found that His guidance at times appeared contrary to the dictates of the Church—as in her ignoring a priest's regulations regarding Catholic burials, or helping poor women avoid the heartbreaking consequences of birthing babies they hadn't the means to care for. In such instances, she followed the dictates of her heart.

Although the sisters were sensitive to Joaquin's need to be alone and gave her the freedom and support to live out her call in her own way, some of them were baffled by it. Hers was not the usual way of a Sisters of Charity nun. In her seeking an eremitic life for almost thirty years, she had become marginal to the Order—as one of her sisters put it, "she was on the fringe, and didn't nurture relations with the Motherhouse."[10] However, the sisters accepted this marginality, and received her back as one of them even after she withdrew from the Order to become a Carmelite. They also respected the fact that she had virtually become a Benedictine during her years at La Soledad and at Christ in the Desert—in practice, if not in vows. Alone in her room her last years at the Motherhouse, she daily recited the psalms of the Hours of the Divine Office at the same times and together in spirit with her Benedictine brothers in their monastery in far-away New Mexico.

The sisters allowed Joaquin to follow her own wishes in dealing with her sickness, and welcomed her back to them with love and compassion at the end of her life. In her desire for the independence to live as she believed was right for her, she stretched her nun's vow of obedience to the limit. This, too, was perhaps indicative of changes in the Catholic order of things over the past forty years. But above all—in her stubborn, prayerful, and independent way—Sister Mary Joaquin always sought to know God's will, and to live her life according to His guidance.

Notes

≈†≈

Part I

Chapter 1

1. Sister Mary Joaquin Bitler papers. (She later changed her name from Mary Joachim to Mary Joaquin.) These papers are in the archives at the Sisters of Charity Motherhouse in Cincinnati, OH. Hereafter reference to these archives will be listed as MJB papers. S/C Archives. The Sisters of Charity were established in Emmitsburg, Maryland in 1809 by Elizabeth Ann Seton, the first American saint (canonized 1975). A few years later, the Emmitsburg group decided to join with the French Daughters of Charity. Some of the sisters felt that this affiliation would not leave them free to respond to the needs of the American Church; hence in 1852 seven of the sisters moved to Ohio and established the community of the Sisters of Charity of Cincinnati. They are a socially active community, managing hospitals and orphanages, teaching in the schools and carrying out other social programs. This is the community of which Sister Mary Joachim was a member.
2. A school for girls, run by the Sisters of Loretto, was established the following year. One of the adobe buildings that would later become the first St. Vincent Hospital was used for a time as a boy's school until a formal school for boys, run by the Christian Brothers of New Orleans, was established in 1859.
3. Laws of the Territory of New Mexico, 16th Session, 1865-66. *An Act to Provide for the Co-operation in the Establishment of the Hospital Lately Erected by the Sisters of Charity.*(See: Angelico Chavez History Library, Santa Fe, NM.

4. The early history of the hospital is recorded in the journal of Sister Catherine Mallon, one of the original four sisters who came to Santa Fe. The journal is in the archives of the Sisters of Charity.

5 Blandina Segale, SC. *At the End of the Santa Fe Trail.* (Albuquerque, NM: University of New Mexico Press, 1932) pp.80 - 81, 112 - 113

6. Clark Kimball and Marcus J. Smith, M.D. *The Hospital at the End of the Santa Fe Trail.* (Santa Fe, NM: Rydal Press, 1977) p.10

7. Miguel Otero. *My Life on the Frontier: 1882 - 1897.* New edition. (Santa Fe, NM: Sunstone Press, 1977) pp.221-222

8. Kimball and Smith, op. cit. p.15

9. *The New Mexican,* July 7, 1970

10. Colorado Fuel and Iron Co. (CF&I), in the early 1900s was owned by John D. Rockefeller, and was the company responsible for Colorado's Ludlow Massacre, 1913 - 1914. The massacre spawned the union activist, Mother Jones

11. Benedicta Mahoney, SC. "We are Many: A History of the Sisters of Charity of Cincinnati, 1898-1971" unpub. ms. 1982, p.165. S/C Archives

12. Information on Sister Mary Joachim's childhood is contained in an unpub. ms. (1970) MJB papers, S/C Archives

13. Giacomo della Chiesa, Cardinal of Bologna, became Pope Benedict XV, 1914 - 1922. He was known as "the peace pope" for his attempts to end the First World War

14. Interview with Benedicta Mahoney, SC, Cincinnati, OH 2008

15. Mary Joachim changed her name to Mary Joaquin around 1970

16. *Santa Fe News,* May 8, 1969

Chapter 2

1. Interview with .Victoria Marie Forde, SC, Cincinnati, OH 2008

2. Interview with Thelma Domenici, Albuquerque, NM 2009. Sister Joachim's music is in the archives of Sisters of Charity

3. Kimball and Smith, op. cit. p.17

4. Ibid.

5. Mahoney, op. cit. p.217

6. Interview with Tom Claffey, Santa Fe, NM 2008

7. *Santa Fe News.* May 8, 1969

8. *The New Mexican.* April 16, 1972

9. Interview with Patrick Marie Bernard, SC. Cincinnati, OH 2008

10. *Our Sunday Visitor.* March 11, 1990

11. MJB papers. Draft article for *Unity*, 1964. S/C Archives

12. Interview with Abe Silver, Santa Fe, NM 2008

13. Interview with Thelma Domenici. Albuquerque, NM. 2009

14. Interview with Mary Ann Getz, Pecos, NM 2008

15. MJB papers. S/C Archives

16. *The New Mexican*. March 21, 1965

17. Ibid. "In Those Days" Retrospective on the Hospital. Jul 11, 1999

18. "She Came, She Saw…" *Northern New Mexico Sunday Magazine*. April 11, 1976

19. *The New Mexican*. April 16. 1972

20. Interview with Dr. Louis Zukal, Santa Fe,NM 2008

21. *The Northern New Mexico Sunday Magazine*, April 11, 1976

22, "Ten Who Made a Difference," *The New Mexican*. November 23, 2006

23. *Santa Fe News*. May 8, 1969

24 "The Vicentian" St. Vincent Hospital Newsletter. December 1972

25. *The New Mexican*. April 11, 1976

26. Interview with John Talley, M.D. Santa Fe, NM 2008

Chapter 3

1. Interview with Lew Thompson. Santa Fe, NM 2008

2. Interview with John Talley, MD. Santa Fe, NM 2008

3. *The New Mexican*. August 27, 1978

4. St. Vincent Hospital. "Newsletter," December, 1972

5. *The New Mexican*. March 21, 1965

6. Information regarding the new St. Vincent Hospital in Santa Fe, NM. 1976. MJB Papers. S/C Archives

7. Interview with Jane Vogt, SC. Cincinnati, OH 2008

8. Interview with Jane Vogt, SC. Cincinnati, OH 2008

Chapter 4

1. "St. Vincent's Master Plan," *The New Mexican*. April 23, 1970

2. St. Vincent Hospital. "Newsletter." December 1972

3. Interview with Jane Vogt, SC. Cincinnati, OH 2008

4. Interview with Lew Thompson. Santa Fe, NM 2008

5. The LPN nursing school, established in 1949, was located in Marian Hall. The

school graduated about three dozen nurses every year
6. Letter from Notre Dame University, granting Sister Joaquin the degree of Master of Industrial Administration. MJB Papers, S/C Archives
7. "The Vicentian." January 1974
8. *The New Mexican.* December 31, 1973

Chapter 5

1. *The New Mexican.* August 27, 1974
2. Interview with Delma Delora, RN. Santa Fe, NM 2008
3. *The New Mexican.* October 13, 1974
4. Ibid. September 12, 1974
5. Ibid. September 13, 1974
6. Ibid.
7. MJB to Mary Assunta Stang, SC. June 18, 1974. S/C Archives.
8. The nurses did not strike; however later in 1988 there was a weeklong walk out, although the nurses promised to cover if there were a major emergency in the area
9. *The New Mexican* July 11, 1975
10. Address given by Seth Montgomery at Sr. Mary Joaquin's retirement dinner. Oct. 1976
11. Interview with Abe Silver. Santa Fe, NM 2008
12. *The New Mexican.* March 23, 1976
13. Ibid. April 11, 1976
14. Ibid. October 19, 1976
15. MJB to John Miriam Jones, SC. January 3, 1995. S/C Archives
16. MJB to Grace Marie Hiltz, SC. June 16, 1972. S/C Archives.
17. Interview with Thelma Domenici. (formerly Sister Ancilla, SC) Albuquerque, NM 2009
18. Raynaud's Phenomenon is a condition resulting in discolorations of the fingers and/or toes in response to changes in temperature—hot or cold—and/ or emotional stress. Initially the fingers/toes turn white from diminished blood supply, then blue because of prolonged lack of oxygen, then the blood vessels reopen, and the blood rushes in turning them red. The phenomenon is often a consequence of rheumatoid arthritis, a progressive autoimmune disease that causes chronic inflammation of the joints and can affect other organs.
19.MJB to Grace Marie Hiltz, SC. April 16, 1976. S/C Archives.

Chapter 6

1. After the 1977 move, Marian Hall stood boarded up for years, occasionally broken into by vandals who apparently stole the hand-carved interior doors. In the 1980s the building was slated for demolition, but was saved by the city's Historical Site Board. The Palace Avenue St. Vincent Hospital building was purchased by the state and served as state offices and a nursing home. In 2009 there are plans to turn both the old hospital building and Marian Hall into a hotel complex.

2. MJB to Regional Superior Mary Christopher Groscheider, SC. July 13, 1976. S/C Archives. Although the Sisters of Charity were no longer involved with St. Vincent's, there were sisters working in other social activities in Santa Fe. The Villa Therese Clinic for the poor, originally opened in 1937, was run by Sisters Patrick Marie Bernard SC, Shirley Le Blanc SC, Margaret Denewith, SC and Dr. Janet Gildea, SC in the 1980s, and other sisters followed. In 1985 a community coalition asked Sister Shirley Le Blanc to start St. Elizabeth's Shelter for the homeless in Santa Fe, with other sisters coming to help over the years. Another Sister of Charity worked in the state penitentiary as a registered pharmacist, and several sisters were working at St. Catherine's Indian School. By 2009, only one Sister of Charity, Sister Juanita Marie Gonzales, is working in Santa Fe, at San Isidro Church, although thirteen are working in Albuquerque and a few in other New Mexico cities.

3. MJB to Mary Assunta Stang, SC, May 10, 1976 S/C Archives. Sister Mary Assunta had worked with Sister Joaquin for a while at St. Vincent's, but left to become president of the Sisters of Charity. Because of her desire for a contemplative life, Mary Joaquin apparently considered the possibility of leaving the Order at this time, but decided against it.

4 MJB to Sr. Mary Assunta Stang, SC, July 19, 1976. S/C Archives. Scleraderma ("hard skin") is a chronic disease, characterized by excessive deposits in the skin and/or other organs. Systemic scleroderma and Raynaud's Phenomenon can cause painful ulcers on the fingers or toes.

5. MJB to Mary Assunta Stang, SC, October 31, 1976. S/C Archives

6.MJB to Annina Morgan, SC. February 7, 1977. S/C Archives

7. MJB to Ken Morrissey. May 10, 1977. S/C Archives

8. MJB to Mary Assunta Stang, SC. February 13, 1977. S/C Archives

9. MJB to Mary Assunta Stang, SC, May 31, 1977. S/C Archives.

10. MJB to Mary Assunta, Stang, SC. Feb 17m 1977 S/C Archives. As a Benedictine monk, Fr. Aelred followed the tenets of the *Rule for Monasteries,* written in the 6th century by Saint Benedict of Nursia. Among many practical

directives for managing the monastery, the *Rule* sets out the Liturgy of the Hours, also called the Hours of the Divine Office, in which specific psalms are chanted at set times beginning in the very early morning and continuing throughout the day.

11. "Some Facts About Your New Hospital." Statement issued by St. Vincent Hospital, 1976

12. Interview with Lew Thompson. Santa Fe, NM 2008

Part II

Chapter 7

1. MJB to Mary Christopher Grosheider, SC, September 24, 1977. S/C Archives

2. MJB Papers Application for Overseas Ministry. Philosophy, and Goals for La Soledad. October 27, 1977. S/C Archives

3. MJB to Annina Morgan, SC. October 27, 1977. S/C Archives

4. S. Eugene Fox. "SC's Hermitage Serves a 'Clinic' for Rural Mexicans." *Intercom*, (November 1981) S/C Archives

5. MJB to Mary Assunta Stang, SC. January 14, 1978. S/C Archives

6. MJB to Mary Assunta Stang, SC. December 30, 1977. *Farolitos* are small candle lanterns, the candles anchored in sand in paper bags. *Luminarias* are bonfires.

7. MJB to Mary Assunta Stang, SC. January 14, 1978. S/C Archives

8. MJB to Mary Assunta Stang, SC. February 19, 1977. S/C Archives

9. MJB to Mary Assunta Stang, SC. February 19, 1977. S/C Archives

10. MJB to Maryanna Coyle, SC. February 27, 1978. S/C Archives

11. MJB. Year-end report and 1979 budget. S/C Archives

12. MJB to Philip Lawrence, OSB. September 1, 1986. Christ in the Desert Archives. (Hereafter C/D Archives)

13. MJB to Mary Assunta Stang, SC. September 28, 1978. S/C Archives

14. Ibid.

Chapter 8

1. MJB to Mary Assunta Stang, SC. September 28, 1978. S/C Archives

2. MJB to Mary Assunta Stang, SC. December 3, 1978. S/C Archives

3. MJB to Mary Assunta Stang, SC. February 3, 1979. S/C Archives

4. MJB to Helen Flaherty, SC. December 3, 1979. S/C Archives

5. MJB to Philip Lawrence, OSB. October 4, 1984. C/D Archives

Chapter 9

1. S. Eugene Fox. op. cit.
2. This is a lose translation of a written statement Luis Brito gave Sister Joaquin. S/C Archives
3. MJB to Philip Lawrence, OSB. October 4, 1984. C/D Archives.
4. MJB to Sisters of Charity. Nov. 25, 1984. S/C Archives.
5. The Christmas, 1985 Newsletter from Rancho La Soledad lists the members of the *Asociación*: Dr. and Mrs. Luis Cervantes, Honorable and Mrs. Pablo López, Mrs. Teresa Lamas, Mrs. Josefina Vásquez, Mrs. María Williams. The Honorable Pablo López was president.
6. Discussion with MJB and the author, Santa Fe, NM, November 1994. One Los Rico woman said that after giving birth to five babies, she went to Sister Joaquin for help. The inoculations kept her infertile until Joaquin left La Soledad, after which she had five more babies. Discussion with Los Rico women and Brother Francisco, April 2009.
7. This story was related to the author by MJB in Santa Fe, NM 1994
8. Deborah Douglas. "Border Crossings." *Weavings: A Journal of the Christian Spiritual Life*. v.17, no.6. (November/December, 2002)
9. MJB to David Douglas. October 24, 1985
10. MJB to David Douglas. November 3, 1985. Brother Francisco recalled later that Florentino made at least fifteen trips to Celaya to get the well permit. He never did get it. Brother Francisco noted that the village has clean well water twenty-four hours a day, which is much more than most rural villagers have still today.
11. MJB to David Douglas. February 24, 1986

Chapter 10

1. Now that electricity has finally come to Los Rico, in 2000 the gasoline pump has been replaced by an electric pump.
2. Today, Waterlines has built more than 700 water projects in underdeveloped countries.
3. "Santa Fe helps Link Mexican Village to the World." *Albuquerque Journal North*, July 15, 1987

4. Conversation with Brother Francisco (Fr. Robert Cumberland) and the author. La Soledad. April 2009

5. The government no longer gives permits to cut the trees in the area.

6. Brother Francisco recalls that Joaquin had about four hours in the morning for prayer and *lectio divina* (spiritual readings) and about the same in the evening. Apparently that did not always seem enough for her

7. Jane Vogt, SC. Papers. S/C Archives.

Chapter 11

1. MJB notes on Dr. Bergere Kenney's funeral. S/C Archives
2. La Soledad "Newsletter." Christmas, 1988
3. MJB letter to donors. Oct 5, 1988. S/C Archives
4. MJB to Philip Lawrence, OSB. July 21, 1989. MCD Archives
5. The hunger program continued until 2005 with an annual budget from Florida's St Maurice Parish including help from Christ in the Desert. The Benedictine nuns were able to help the children and the elderly of the village at an average cost of 27 cents per person per day.
6. Denise Kusel. "The Hermit Who Changed Healthcare." *The New Mexican* July 11, 1990
7. The letters quoted in this book are almost entirely letters *from* Sister Joaquin to others who saved them; a very few are from copies made of letters sent to her. Most are in the S/C Archives or the C/D Archives
8. An indult is permission from the Congregation of Religious and Secular Institutes in the Vatican for a religious to change from one order to another. The indult for Sister Mary Joaquin was not approved until the 30th of December, although she entered the Carmelite monastery on December 8. The Carmelite Order was established in the 13th century, and women, always cloistered, were included in the Order in the 15th. Two of the most famous Carmelites, active in the Reformation Period, were St. Teresa of Avila and the poet St. John of the Cross
9. MJB papers. S/C Archives
10. Conversation with MJB and the author. Santa Fe, NM 1994

Part III

Chapter 12

1. Susan H. Kelly.Conversation with MJB. Santa Fe, NM 1994
2. MJB to Philip Lawrence,OSB August 18, 1989. C/D Archives
3. *Intercom*. March 1990
4. MJB to John Miriam Jones, SC. January 3, 1995. S/C Archives
5. "Que Pasa?" St. Vincent Hospital Newsletter. December 21, 1990
6.Seth Montgomery. Statement in honor of MJB. Santa Fe, NM July 25, 1991
7. In 1998, the contractor, Burke Denman, received the Renew America Green Building and Real Estate Development Award for the environmentally sensitive work at the monastery. See: Mari Graña, *Brothers of the Desert*. (Santa Fe, NM: Sunstone Press, 2006) pp.123-124
8. MJB to Grace Ann Gratsch, SC. November 14, 1998. S/C Archives.
9. MJB to John Miriam Jones, SC. January 15 and 16, 1994. S/C Archives.

Chapter 13

1. Marguerite Claffey's grandfather, T. D. Burns, once owned the Spanish land grant in the Chama Canyon where the Monastery of Christ in the Desert is now located.
2. MJB to Grace Ann Gratsch, SC. November 27, 1999. S/C Archives.
3. Interview with Jane Vogt, SC. November 2008

Epilogue

1. For a time there was the psychiatric hospital in Santa Fe, Piñon Hills. It closed a few years after St. Vincent's opened its 37-bed psychiatric unit in 1985.
2. The Stark Law (Third Amendment, 2007) prohibits physicians from referring Medicare patients to hospitals and other entities with which they have a financial relationship, unless the arrangement fits into one of a number of specific exceptions. "What do I need to know about the Stark III Rules?" *Massachusetts Medical Law Report*, June 15, 2008)
3. *Business Wire*. May 22, 2007

4. See: christushealth.org/about_main.htm
5. *The New Mexican*, Jan 9, 2009. According to CEO Valdez, elective abortions and sterilizations can be performed at a community facility close to the hospital.
6. "Hospital Merger Goes into Effect" *Albuquerque Journal Santa Fe.* April 10, 2008
7. *The New Mexican*, May 2, 2009
8. Fr. Robert Cumberland (Brother Francisco) to author. May 3, 2009
9. Ibid
10. Interview with Patrick Marie Bernard, SC. Cincinnati.OH. November, 2008

Acknowledgements

≈†≈

I am grateful to the many Sisters of Charity of Cincinnati, Ohio for discussing with me their friendship with Sister Mary Joaquin, especially to Sister Judith Metz, SC and Sister Benedicta Mahoney, SC, who provided me access to the Motherhouse archives of St. Vincent Hospital and to Sister Joaquin's papers. Sister Judith took time out to help me from her planning for the Sisters of Charity celebration in 2009 of two hundred years of service in the United States and many other countries. I want to acknowledge the members of the Santa Fe Writers' Group, who reviewed the manuscript many times over. I also want to acknowledge the help of the doctors, nurses, and volunteers who worked at Saint Vincent Hospital in Santa Fe. Jean Marr of the St. Vincent Hospital Auxiliary opened the auxiliary's historical scrapbooks to me. I am especially grateful to Father Robert Cumberland (Brother Francisco), who accompanied me to La Soledad in April 2009. Father Cumberland related to me the history of the local area and translated the stories and comments of the villagers of Los Rico, who remember Sister Joaquin with great love. I also want to thank Father Ezequiel Bas Luna and Brother Fernando Hool Salazar and their brother monks for their gracious hospitality at the Monastery of La Soledad. I also wish to thank Father Christian Leisy, OSB of the Monastery of Christ in the Desert who made the monastery's archives of Sister Joaquin's letters available to me, and to Abbot Philip Lawrence, OSB of the monastery, who graciously and promptly answered my many emails. I appreciate the help from many of Sister Joaquin's Santa Fe friends: especially Peggy Jones who related many stories of her good friend; Susan H. Kelly and Lew Thompson; and David and Deborah Douglas, who lent me their files on the water well adventure and graciously let me use their photographs. Tom Claffey offered me many personal reminiscences of the Sister he considered as a sister of his own. Lastly, I thank the villagers of Los Rico, who recounted many stories of "Madrecita."

People Interviewed

~†~

Sr. Jane Vogt, SC. Cincinnati, OH
Sr. Celestia Koebel, SC. Cincinnati, OH
Sr. Patrick Marie Bernard, SC. Cincinnati, OHSC
Sr. Victoria Marie Forde, SC. Cincinnati, OH
Sr. Benedicta Mahoney SC. Cincinnati, OH
Sr. Judith Metz, SC. Archivist, Cincinnati, OH
Luis Zukal, M.D. Santa Fe, NM
John Talley M.D. Santa Fe, NM
Grant La Farge, M.D. Santa Fe, NM
William Jones, M.D. Santa Fe, NM
Peggy Jones. Santa Fe, NM
David Douglas. Santa Fe, NM
Deborah Douglas. Santa Fe, NM
Delma Delora, RN. Santa Fe, NM
Mary Karsis, RN. Santa Fe, NM
Rita Giugliotti, RN. Santa Fe, NM
Joe Valdes, Sr. Santa Fe, NM
Tom Claffey. Santa Fe, NM
Mary Ann Getz. Pecos, NM
Susan Rush. Santa Fe, NM
Abe Silver. Santa Fe, NM

Marian Silver. Santa Fe, NM
Thelma Domenici. Albuquerque, NM
David Kenney. Albuquerque, NM
Owen Lopez. Santa Fe, NM
Richard Polese. Santa Fe, NM
Lew Thompson. Santa Fe, NM
Laughlin Barker. Santa Fe, NM
Susan H. Kelly. Santa Fe, NM
Jean Marr. St. Vincent Hospital Auxiliary, Santa Fe, NM
Abbot Philip Lawrence, OSB. Abiquiú, NM
Fr. Christian Leisy, OSB. Abiquiú, NM
Fr. Robert Cumberland. Arteaga, Mexico
Fr. Ezequiel Bas Luna, OSB. La Soledad, Mexico
Br. Fernando Hool Salazar, OSB. La Soledad, Mexico
Sr. Juanita Marie Gonzales, SC. Santa Fe, NM

LaVergne, TN USA
13 September 2010
196782LV00006B/12/P